Re-Reading Altschul

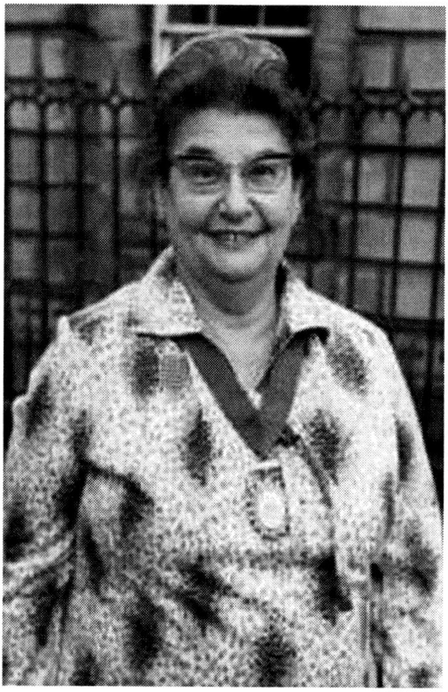

Annie Altschul

Re-Reading Altschul
A Festchrift

In honour of the late
Professor Emeritus Annie Altschul
CBE, BA, MSc, RGN, RMN, RNT

The Hypatia Trust
Penzance
2004

First published in 2004 by
The Hypatia Trust
Trevelyan House
16 Chapel Street
Penzance
Cornwall TR18 4AW

Typeset in-house in Adobe Garamond. Design by Phil Budden.
Printed in Great Britain by Pims, Basildon, Essex

ISBN 1 872229 52 2

Contents

Annie Therese Altschul (1919-2001)

Annie departed Vienna in 1938 for London at the age of 19, as the tensions in Europe threatened to explode. She trained as a general nurse and midwife at Epsom County Hospital, followed by becoming a student in the therapeutic community formed by Dr Maxwell Jones at the Army mental hospital at Mill Hill, a war-time outpost for the Maudsley Hospital. In the move from Mill Hill back to the Royal Bethlem and Maudsley Hospital in South London, she professed disappointment in the way that the staff 'forgot everything they had learned at Mill Hill. They returned to pre-war methods.'

In 1948 she completed a nurse tutor's course, and began to build her influential reputation as a psychiatric nurse-thinker. In 1952, by attending evening classes, she was one of the first people to graduate with an internal London University degree in psychology. *Aids to Psychiatric Nursing* (1957) and *Psychology for Nurses* (1962) preceded her move in 1964 to become a lecturer in the Department of Nursing Studies at Edinburgh University. In 1976 she became the second-ever Professor of Nursing Studies following on from her friend and colleague, Margaret Scott Wright. Her major and seminal work *Patient-Nurse Interaction* (1972), like her previous texts, has been re-issued and revised, to become a classic work.

Mathematics, music and multiple friendships were her life-long avocations. She was a down-to-earth woman with no pretensions and little time for pride in her accomplishments or her honours, though they were many. Her gift to us, as so many are aware, is that of *relationship* – to work, to knowledge, to ourselves, and to each other. This book is a small but worthy tribute to that fact.

Melissa Hardie, 2004

Foreword

It is an honour to have been invited to contribute this foreword to the proceedings of the Festschrift held in honour of Annie Altschul – and in which she participated – shortly before her death in December 2001.

While I never had the privilege of meeting Professor Altschul, I am well aware of her outstanding body of work and her distinguished position in mental health nursing both worldwide and in the UK. I can certainly relate to her focus on mental health nursing, as it is such an important foundation of my own nursing career and practice.

Despite having officially retired many years ago, Annie Altschul has remained an important personality in nursing in the United Kingdom and indeed internationally. Not only for her distinguished career, but for the profoundly important impact she has had on patient care and on nursing, and for her warmth of personality.

Undoubtedly her own life experiences contributed to her nursing perspective, for example her flight, as a young Jewish woman, from the Nazi threat to refuge then permanent residence in the United Kingdom. It surely contributed to her delicate cultural sensitivity when she spent a year in the USA in the early 1960s looking at mental health nursing.

As a nurse from the US, I am proud that she found many positives in our attitudes to patient care and nursing education in those distant days. That she also found US nurses to be so candid about the challenges and problems surely reflects the mature and non-judgemental way in which she engaged with them.

Annie Altschul's work will continue to have a positive impact on the quality of care in mental health nursing for a long time to come. She accumulated many honours during her lifetime for her influential work in education and research, yet she never lost sight of the central importance of the therapeutic relationship between patient and nurse, something which she shared with Hildegard Peplau whom I am privileged to call my mentor.

I understand that Annie wore her many academic and public honours, including her RCN Fellowship, very lightly. I agree that the focus should always be on the achievement that has merited the honour, rather than the honour itself. But I also believe that the honours Annie received say some important things about the way in which our society and the nursing profession have come to perceive mental health.

We know that one in four people will be affected by mental ill health at some time in their life. This stark statistic proves that we simply cannot afford to continue to stigmatise people suffering in this way, or to marginalise those who care for them. Public honours like those that Annie Altschul received have helped bring mental health issues into the mainstream.

As a profession, nursing deserves to be judged by its treatment of newcomers – but also by the way it supports and celebrates individuals who have made a significant contribution to nursing. I believe that we are getting it right with Annie Altschul. We have used and celebrated her contributions during her lifetime and we are taking them forward with us into the future through endeavours such as this publication. I commend it to you.

Beverly Malone

General Secretary of the Royal College of Nursing.

Preface

Annie planned carefully for her death. One of the things she did was to go through her papers and convey them to others. The main part of these she gave to the Royal College of Nursing archives, through Susan McGann, the RCN archivist. On one occasion she asked me to take some papers to Susan, and said that I could read them first if I wished, as they related to her visit to the United States in 1960-61 and she knew I was interested in her part in mediating British and American psychiatric nursing discourses (Tilley 1999).

I read the papers with great interest and fascination. Here, I thought, were primary documents relating to a key moment in the history of British psychiatric nursing. They gave an account of what she sought in the U.S., what she found, and what she did not find which she considered important. Importantly for me, they gave insight into the origins of the MSc dissertation, published as *Patient- Nurse Interaction* (Altschul 1972), analysis of which has been the focus of my PhD dissertation and a long-running conversation or 'argument' between Annie and myself. The most fascinating documents, for me, were those relating to her time in Boston, her one-to-one relationship with a patient, and her relationship with her supervisor in Boston, June Mellow. For me, as a teacher, who had taken Annie's work as touchstone for understanding psychiatric nursing when a student, these accounts of her own role of student and 'speaking up' to her teacher/supervisor, were like gold.

I knew these works needed the widest possible readership among nursing practitioners, students, teachers and researchers, not only as historical documents but as living testimony to a great nurse's powers of observation, criticism, and love of those whom she served and from whom she learned. They were also the best expression of Annie's complex character I had read.

I mooted first with Annie, then with Susan McGann and Barbara Mortimer and colleagues in the Department of Nursing Studies where Annie was Professor Emeritus, whether the papers might form the basis for a celebration of her life and work. A celebration was timely, as Annie reminded us often that she was making no plans for the future. She was engaging with the process of helping me and others get used to the fact she was dying.

I got together a team of contributors who knew Annie and whose views would give a sense of the spectrum of responses the papers might occasion. Each had something invaluable and unique to contribute. I will not detail this as their own papers do that better than I could. David Glenister gave me the key term - '*festschrift*', reminding us that it was most appropriate to its purpose because of Annie's own linguistic origins. The title of the 17th November 2001 event, a one-day celebration of Annie Altschul's contribution to psychiatric nursing - past, present and future, was 'Re-reading Altschul: A Festschrift in Honour of Professor Emeritus Annie Altchul CBE BA MSc RGN RMN RNT FRCN'.

Susan McGann played a vital role in offering the RCN's premises, financial and administrative support for the occasion, and in planning and printing Annie's papers for the event. Barbara Mortimer took a major role in planning the day's event, and in developing the web version of this publication. Professors Kath Melia and Alison Tierney in the School of Nursing Studies, University of Edinburgh, helped organise support, to include a financial contribution from the Sheila Allan bequest. Numerous others contributed individually and collectively to making the occasion a success. On the day some 25 people gathered in a setting familiar to Annie. They had been sent and asked to read her papers in advance so they could take part in the conversation about them, with Annie and each other. In the morning session, they listened and responded to the six papers written for the discussion, including Annie's introduction. In the afternoon, we all became a 'big group', discussing Annie's U.S. visit, her work, and the views of the presenters. Many in the group made rich contributions to an occasion for engagement with, response to, and appreciation of Annie's work and life.

Jack Shea, a documentary film maker, filmed the *festschrift*. Therefore, we have a visual record of the event. This publication is another document, another contribution to the play of texts, readings, responses, which Annie loved and at which she was *'il miglior fabbro'*.

Melissa Hardie, a former senior research fellow and Ph.D. in Nursing Studies at Edinburgh, responded enthusiastically to my request for help in publishing this paperback version of the Festschrift proceedings. Her company, Patten Press (now Hypatia Publications) previously published Sheila Allan's biography of Elsie Stephenson, the founder of the Nursing Studies Unit at the University of Edinburgh: *Fear Not to Sow*, and I believed it especially fitting that this tribute to Annie's own work should follow suit. Allan wrote that she had 'recalled the uniquely personal relationship between staff and students [in the Department of Nursing Studies and in Edinburgh University], a tradition which Elsie had firmly established. I mentioned to the Professor [Annie] how much the extracts of the Elsie Stephenson Collection had affected me, and how I would love to be involved in piecing together a biography of Elsie. "Why don't you do it then?" she asked. Why indeed?' (Allan 1990, p. vi)

I wonder whether, and in what ways, the 'tradition' of 'the uniquely personal relationship between students and staff' at Edinburgh was informed by Annie's sojourn in America, and the relationships she formed there with patients, students and staff, particularly at Boston University. It would be fitting indeed if, through the wider readership this book enables, a kindred spirit were spurred to involvement in 'piecing together a biography' of Annie.

The 'Bibliography' in this volume was compiled mainly by Clare Soutby-Tailyour, then an Honours student in Nursing Studies at the University of Edinburgh; with additional bibliographical material compiled by David Glenister, School of Nursing, University of Hull. It is not complete, with no entries after 1999. It is a remarkable (and characteristic) fact that the last of Annie's publications of which I am aware - Altschul, Annie T (2002) – appeared after her death, and 112 pages after her obituary! In many ways, then, her words have lived and will live after her. I especially hope that students of this and future generations will be stimulated, provoked, encouraged by the texts in this volume to read more of Annie's work, and hear as addressed to them Annie's spirited challenge to argument.

A note, too, on editing. I do not know whether the reports Annie gave me to convey to the RCN Archives were exact copies of the final versions, or whether she edited them at some later stage. The texts were scanned for publication for the *festschrift*; inevitably some minor changes to the text resulted, which Susan McGann and I tried to pick up at that stage. Barbara Mortimer and I did further minor editing / proofreading to produce the web version. That version I have re-proofed against the original texts. I settled on a (perhaps) idiosyncratic editorial strategy, aimed at keeping as close as possible to Annie's original text. Annie's style was distinctive and eminently clear; nonetheless marked by e.g. occasional variation in use of commas, and in usage (e.g. she wrote 'one to one relationship' rather than the now-conventional 'one-to-one relationship'. Where I thought it obvious that Annie would have corrected something, I have done so; where e.g. a word seems to be missing I have added it in brackets. A main reason I have adopted a conservative approach in editing is that I want students to see, as near as I can render it, Annie's work as she wrote it when moved by passion or desire to speak directly, to teacher or funder, or unwittingly, to these students themselves.

Steve Tilley

Senior Lecturer, Nursing Studies
University of Edinburgh
31 Buccleuch Place
Edinburgh EH8 9JT
Scotland

References:

Allan, S. (1990) *Fear Not To Sow: A Life of Elsie Stephenson.* Jamieson Library and Patten Press, Penzance.

Altschul, A. (1972) *Patient-Nurse Interaction*, Churchill Livingstone, Edinburgh.

Tilley, S. (1999) 'Altschul's legacy in mediating British and American psychiatric nursing discourses: common sense and the 'absence' of the accountable practitioner'. *Journal of Psychiatric and Mental Health Nursing*, 6 (4) 283-296.

Paper 1

Itinerary of a tour of USA, Canada, and Australia, to study psychiatric nursing

Annie Altschul

May 1960 – April 1961 **Programme of study visits**

1-8 May, 1960	American Nursing Association (ANA) Convention, Miami Beach
9-11 May	American Psychiatric Association Convention, Atlantic City
12-18 May	New York City: Meetings with ANA Officers, National League of Nurses, American Nurses Foundation
19-22 May	Chicago: Visits to Child Guidance Clinics

23 May – 23 August: California

23-24 May	Sacramento: Discussion with staff at State Department of Mental Hygiene
25-27 May	San Francisco: Langley Porter Clinic (Adult & Child Psychiatric Clinic, Medical Centre of University of San Francisco); Psychiatric Department of School of Nursing of University of San Francisco; Discussion with Miss Kalkman
1-3 June	Porterville Hospital (for mental subnormality)
4-25 June	Camarillo Hospital (for mental Illness in adults and children): Special Unit for Adolescents. *The largest hospital I visited.*

7 June	Visit to Bakersfield Junior College: 2-year Associate Arts Degree in Nursing
28-30 June	Norwalk Hospital, near Los Angeles (for mentally ill)
5-6 July	Napa Hospital (for mentally ill)
7-8 July	Sonoma Hospital (for mentally retarded)
11-13 July	Mendocino Hospital (for mentally ill)
14-17 July	Sacramento State Department
18-20 July	De Witt Hospital (for mentally ill)
21-22 July	San Francisco: Langley Porter Clinic
25 July	San Joaquin: Stockton Community Clinic
26-29 July	San Francisco: Public Health Department; University of California (Berkeley)
1-3 August	San Mateo Community Clinic
4-6 August	Sacramento State Department
8-10 August	Pacific State Hospital (for mentally subnormal)
11-12 August	Fairview Hospital (for mentally subnormal)
15-18 August	Atascadero Hospital (for criminally insane and sexual psychopaths)
23-25 August	Oregon: Salem Hospital (for mentally ill)
5-9 September	New York: Discussions with ANA

12 September – 18 December: Boston, Massachusetts
[Enrolled at Boston University School of Nursing - Clinical work at Massachusetts Mental Health Centre]

4-7 November	Hartford, Connecticut: State Hospital (*to see re-motivation*)
11 November	Austin Riggs Private Mental Hospital

16 November	Massachusetts Memorial Hospital: psychiatric ward in General Hospital
9 December	Hartford: State Department of Mental Hygiene. Meeting with nursing instructors from all hospitals, including Institute of Living
14 December	Worcester, Mass: State Hospital
16 December	McLean Hospital

Other visits during this time: several to Boston State Hospital

Discussions with Mrs Lenahan, State Department of Mental Health

Visits to Harvard University School of Public Health

Discussion with School of Education lecturers, Boston University, concerning Boston experiments with juvenile delinquency prevention

Meeting with Dr Gerald Caplan, concerning techniques of consultation

19-22 December: Chicago, Illinois

19 December	Chicago: Cook County Hospital (Receiving Hospital for all emergency admissions for the city). *I was present at legal commitments on that day.*
20 December	Illinois State Psychiatric Institute
21-22 December	Psychiatric Clinic, University of Chicago

27 December - 14 January 1961: Iowa City, Iowa

Based at University of Iowa School of Nursing

9 January	Des Moines State Department of Mental Health (discussion on State Board Examinations for nurses)
10 January	Clarinda Hospital (for mentally ill)
13-14 January	Mount Pleasant Hospital (for mentally ill)

16-19 January: Baltimore, Maryland

Johns Hopkins Research Institutes

Phipps Clinic

Rosewood Hospital and Training School for the Retarded

23-31 January: Washington, D.C.

23 January	Esther Garrison, Training Specialist, National Institutes of Health, Welfare and Education (NIH)
24 January	Chestnut Lodge (Private Mental Hospital)
25 January	Margaret Arnstein. Public Health Service, Nursing Studies
26 January	Clinical Centre, NIH
27 January	NI Mental Health, meeting with staff from St. Elizabeth's Hospital
30 January	Lucile P. Leone, Chief Nursing Officer, Office of Surgeon General

1-25 February: New York & New Jersey

1-3 February	Presbyterian Hospital, NY
6-8 February	Manhattan State Hospital
9-10 February	Teachers College, NY

13-15 February	NY State Psychiatric Institute
16 February	Manhattan Veterans Hospital
17 February	Albany: Montefiore Hospital (Psychiatric ward & day hospital)
18-20 February	Albany: NY State Department of Mental Hygiene; Hudson State Hospital
21 February	Skidmore College (NY) School of Nursing
22-23 February	New York University
27 February	Bronx Community College (2 yr course) Trenton State Hospital, New Jersey
28 February	Lyons Veterans Hospital, New Jersey

1-10 March: Canada

Visits to Montreal General Hospital (psychiatric ward); Allan Memorial Clinic;

McGill University; Ottawa;

Canadian Registered Nurses Association;

Toronto Psychiatric Clinic

New Toronto Psychiatric Hospital

15-16 March: Hawaii

Hawaii State Mental Hospital

20 March - 26 April: Australia

Royal Newcastle Hospital

Callan Park Mental Hospital, Sydney

Broughton Hall Psychiatric Hospital, Sydney

Ryde Mental Hospital, Sydney

Royal Park, Melbourne

International Congress of Nursing

27 April: Singapore

Woodbridge Hospital, Singapore

Paper 2

Report on a tour of the United States of America, Canada, and Australia, to study psychiatric nursing, May 1960-April 1961

A. Altschul B.A., S.R.N., R.M.N., S.T.D.

[Report to the Commonwealth Fund]

This is, of necessity, a very brief report of an exceedingly full and profitable year spent in the United States of America, Canada and Australia. The trip was made possible through the generosity of the British Commonwealth for Nurses Scholarship Fund, who awarded me a scholarship in 1959, the Board of Governors of the Bethlem Royal Hospital and the Maudsley Hospital and the S.E. Metropolitan Area Nurse Training Committee who granted me a year's leave, and helped to finance the journey. I enclose a list of hospitals and other agencies I visited, and will later prepare a detailed account of all that I believe to be of special interest to us in this country.

It is not possible or appropriate to give details of all the many people whose acquaintance I made during the year and who offered me hospitality, friendship and a host of memorable experiences. I should, however, like to thank them all here and to stress how much the private enjoyment has contributed towards the professional experience. It is, of course, impossible to understand the significance of a people's attitude to work, to sickness and to the profession without a love of its culture. Living in the U.S.A. for nearly a year meeting people in their own homes, meeting their families, sharing with them leisure and work, enjoyment and anxieties, has helped me to understand a little more about the U.S.A. than I had done before. I met people in all walks of life, rich and poor, white and coloured, young and old, intelligent and stupid. I met many people in no way connected with nursing and learnt a little about the way they view their health services and the nursing profession. I met doctors and other health workers, and nurses of all kinds - ranging from the newest students to those in top level executive positions, professional nurses, auxiliary nursing personnel, hospital staff and public health nurses, faculty and students in University and in hospital schools.

Meeting so many different people can be a confusing experience. Having formed some conclusion about the U.S.A., these promptly had to be revised in the light of new experiences. However, there is no short and simple way to knowing so large and complex a country as the U.S.A. I am profoundly grateful that I was able to spend so long in the U.S.A., and that I never felt I had to hurry. Time and time again when I stayed several days in the same hospitals I gained information during the last day of my stay only because during the early part my hosts and myself had had time to relax, to know each other well and to trust each other. I could not help reflecting on the arrangements I have seen for some of our overseas visitors and for some English nurses in the U.S.A. Whilst congratulating myself on my good fortune in having arranged a leisurely trip, I should like to make a plea to all who are concerned with arrangements of tours, to allow for fewer and longer visits. I should like to thank Miss Rowe and Miss Selby-Lownes for their help and Miss Deane for her part in smoothing my way on this side of the Atlantic.

My thanks are due to the American Nurses Association for their invitation to the Convention, and for arranging observation visits in New York, Washington and Baltimore. To the American Nurses Foundation, and particularly to Dr. Hardin, for giving me so much interesting information, allowing me to browse and for all the helpful suggestions. To the many nurses in the National League of Nurses for discussing with me nursing policy, standards, examinations and many other topics.

I am grateful to the Dean and faculty of Boston University School of Nursing for accepting me as a student and helping me to understand nursing education.

Most of all I should like to thank Mrs. K. Steele, Director of Nursing Services in the State Department of Mental Hygiene, for the tremendous help she has given me during the 3 months stay in California. Her constant help and support, her advice, and her introduction to nurses in other State Departments were of inestimable value to me. I should also like to thank her and Dr. Blain for doing me the honour of inviting me to serve as training consultant to the California State hospitals. I hope that they found their trust in me justified. For me it was of tremendous value to be invited into the hospitals, to be so warmly received and so completely accepted during my stay in California.

While I do not wish to detract in any way from the value contact with the A.N.A. has been to me, I should like to emphasise the advantages of contact with State Departments of Mental Health for any nurses who wish to gain information about psychiatric nursing in the United States. My own initial contacts were with the State Department of California, and thanks to Mrs. Steele I met nurses in the State Departments of New York, Massachusetts, Connecticut, Iowa, New Jersey and Washington all of whom were extremely helpful.

My first week in the USA was spent at Miami Beach, observing and participating in the Convention of the A.N.A. This was a very stimulating experience. The number of nurses present alone, made it a most impressive Convention. There were so many meetings going on simultaneously that it was difficult to choose the most interesting and worth while.

During my later visits to schools of nursing, in the U.SA. I came to appreciate more fully the value of having listened to American nurses discussing their profession right at the beginning of the tour Quite frequently, later, when I was inclined to be critical of nursing practice or nursing education, it was good to remember how seriously American nurses criticised themselves and how many different opinions I had heard expressed about every conceivable professional topic, during the week in Miami Beach.

When I first tried to formulate my aims and objectives, I put very high on the list my desire to find out how psychiatric nursing was incorporated in the basic comprehensive nursing course. Internationally a comprehensive training appears to be the aim and there are many people in this country who would like to see the end of the General Nursing Council's separate registers for Mental Nurses. Instead, they would like to see the student prepared in a comprehensive training for first level positions in all branches of nursing.

I had myself been concerned with providing students in general nursing with a short experience in the psychiatric hospitals. Having had serious doubts about the value of this, and no idea at all about the best way to introduce the student to psychiatry, I had hoped that in the United States, where this was no new idea, I would find clearly defined aims, well planned curricula, and sound evaluation of the psychiatric experience.

In order to study specifically the psychiatric affiliations, I felt the need to acquaint myself with many other aspects of nursing and mental health in the U.SA.

It was necessary to find out what provisions there were for the mentally ill, both in institutions and in the community, how mental health and mental illness were viewed by the public in general, the patients, their relatives, and professional people in particular. The care of the mentally ill and the education of the people who provided care had to be looked at. Nursing education as a whole, not only its psychiatric aspects, had to be understood. To evaluate basic nursing education, it became necessary to learn something about the provisions for post graduate studies, the career opportunities in nursing and the problems relating to inter-professional tensions between nurses and other health workers.

Nursing education cannot be properly understood without some idea of the general educational ideals and practices in the U.S.A., and nursing cannot be viewed without a knowledge of the people's expectations of and attitudes to doctors, hospitals and health services.

My terms of reference became so wide that obviously a year was not enough to answer all my questions. My initial problem, the integration of psychiatry into the comprehensive nursing training was the one which in the end received least illumination, and I became increasingly interested in the education of those people who gave nursing care to patients. but who were not, in fact, nurses - people called aides, or attendants, or technicians in different states!

A year turned out to be too short a time to learn enough about nursing in the U.S.A. It is, however, I believe, the maximum time during which I personally could have remained sufficiently detached to be a visitor and so gain the kind of information I was seeking. If I had stayed any longer, I would have become involved in nursing problems and could have felt that I belonged to the U.S.A.

A year, I think, is also almost too long to try and remember what conditions are like in one's own country and to compare objectively what one sees with what one remembers. I found it very hard at times to prevent my memory playing tricks on me.

Towards the end of the year, I could only remember the best of what I had known in Great Britain and even that took on a rose-coloured hue. I had to remind myself, quite forcefully, that I had found plenty to criticise in this country, and that my desire to travel had been fostered by my discontent with conditions as they were.

Throughout my stay in the U.S.A. I attempted to visit hospitals which had something of value to offer, and to talk to people who were well informed and had new ideas for the future. I did not go out of my way to see the worst. On the other hand, my American hosts made no attempt ever to restrict my visits to showplaces. They allowed me free access to all their facilities, invited me to all their discussions and conferences, and, frequently, deliberately showed me those aspects of their provisions about which they were most worried or concerned. In all I believe I saw a very fair cross section of hospitals and clinics and spoke to a very representative sample of people.

Perhaps the most startling difference between American nurses and British nurses is the easy unembarrassed way in which American nurses allowed me to see not only what they thought good, but also what they thought bad, the way they included me in discussions and meetings in which their shortcomings or their staff problems were being discussed.

I spent approximately one-third of my time in the U.S.A. in California, as the guest of the State Department of Mental Hygiene. During this time I visited 6 mental hospitals, 4 hospitals for the retarded, 1 University clinic and 2 community clinics. I spent considerable time discussing mental health problems with the staff of the Department of Mental Hygiene, with nurses at the Public Health Department, and with Members of the faculty of the University of California in San Francisco.

My main interests were in the provisions for the mentally ill under the Short-Doyle legislation, in the standards of care in the hospitals I visited, and in the in-service training programmes for all the staff in the hospitals.

About one-third of my time was spent at Boston University where I enrolled as a special student in the School of Nursing. There I had the opportunity to gain first-hand knowledge of Masters and Doctoral courses in psychiatric nursing. I had the opportunity to meet student nurses from a variety of schools, to participate in the clinical experience of students and to gain experience of University life in the U.S.A. During this time I paid particular attention to nursing research, particularly in the psychiatric field.

The rest of my stay in the U.S.A. was spent on observation visits of short duration to hospitals and schools of nursing in Chicago, Iowa, New York, Baltimore, Washington D.C., New Jersey and Hawaii. During this time I tried to get a varied picture and to see especially places which were in some way unusual or even unique.

At the end of my tour I spent a short time in Canada, too short to appreciate the special features of Canadian psychiatric problems. I had a very interesting time in all the hospitals I visited, and would like to take the opportunity of thanking all concerned, and particularly Miss McColl, for the arrangements and for their hospitality.

In Australia I visited several hospitals in Sydney and Melbourne, and on my return journey I spent a most enjoyable morning in the Woodbridge Hospital, Singapore.

Every one of the hospitals and schools I visited deserves a detailed description and evaluation. In this report it is only possible to give an overall view, and to discuss some of the general observations and conclusions.

Community Care

There is a growing awareness among professional people in the U.S.A. of the need to decentralise mental treatment. In some areas, particularly in the West, psychiatrists believe it to be better for the patient to be treated outside mental hospitals, but this is not a universal opinion. Many analytically orientated psychiatrists treat their patients in hospital for long periods when hospitalisation as such did not appear to me to be of benefit.

However, an attempt to stop the building of large hospitals and to provide a variety of local clinics and treatment facilities is gaining popularity.

In the past there have been few enormously large mental hospitals - the largest I visited has 8,500 beds; there are larger ones. Patients and their relatives travel hundreds of miles and obviously it is impossible, under such conditions, to provide effective aftercare, to give help to the family or to encourage the patient to maintain contact.

Decentralisation and provisions for community care take many forms. I have seen day hospitals, psychiatric wards attached to general hospitals, out-patient facilities and special clinics for alcoholics.

Public Health Nurses are becoming increasingly concerned with their role in psychiatric work, and are studying psychiatric nursing in post-graduate courses. They are involved in research projects, attempting to see what help they can give before, during and after a mental illness. Psychiatric nurses are being used as consultants by public health nurses, and there are some interesting projects to help psychiatric nurses to learn the principles of consultation. Dr. Gerald Caplan in Boston in particular has developed this idea.

Psychiatric social workers on the other hand do not appear to concern themselves at all with the community or the social effects of psychiatric illness. They prefer to do "case work" with individual patients or to conduct group therapy. I found it difficult to distinguish their function from that of the psychiatrist or the psychologist.

Community provisions depend to some extent on special legislation being passed. This is necessary to provide the money and also to make it possible to provide treatment without recourse to the usual laws. In California the Short-Doyle Act has made it possible for the local communities to plan psychiatric facilities in connection with the community hospitals.

I saw two such clinics. These are centres for out-patients, and are responsible for education of the public as well as providing in-patient facilities.

The ward in San Mateo was one of the most interesting units I visited. It is in some ways similar to an observation ward in this country in that it has to accept all emergency admissions. About one-third of the patients remain in the ward for up to 90 days for treatment, the others are transferred to other hospitals within a few days. It was amazing to see the improvement effected in a very short time as a result of the wonderful atmosphere of the ward, the enthusiasm of all the staff - medical and nursing, and their very high degree of skill.

Group therapy was used and all the staff were kept fully informed. All doctors were present at morning report, all staff met during the morning, and all details of treatment were fully discussed. The ward was open and patients acted as receptionists and kept the door under observation. The kitchen was freely accessible to all patients, who made coffee and helped themselves to nourishment from the refrigerator.

Nurses did not wear uniform.

Many of these features were observed in other hospitals too. I mention it here because it impressed me, particularly in view of the very serious disturbance of all the patients on admission and the tremendous improvement observed.

The problem of involving the community more in the treatment of patients and organising quicker discharge and better follow up is highly complex. It is different in each state, partly because of the geography, partly because of the different laws which apply in each state to the compulsory detention of patients, partly because the provisions of mental health services are intimately connected with politics. Each state approaches its problems differently, but the deep concern about the problem is universal.

On the whole I thought the laws relating to mental disorder restrictive. States vary in the extent to which they adhere to application of their own laws and in some states, patients are being admitted without formality to wards in general hospitals or to day hospitals.

The extent to which politics enter into decisions about the care of the sick was a surprise to me. Many professional appointments are made on political grounds and changes in staff follow on the election of a new Governor. This affects planning of all the facilities for the mentally ill, but in particular, community care.

Mental Hospitals

I saw a very large number of hospitals, all of which were newer than most hospitals in this country, some were brand new or not even completed. Hospitals are generally much larger than we would consider desirable. The very large ones are not favoured by the Americans themselves, but they apparently do not consider 3,000 beds too large, and are constructing wards for 60 patients even now.

On the whole, bedroom facilities are good. bed spacing better than in many English hospitals. A lot of attention is paid to kitchens and dining rooms.

All hospitals have excellent gardens, in every hospital attempts are made to provide hairdressing facilities and washing machines. All patients have access to iced drinks, coffee and tea at all times.

The day rooms are small, overcrowded, uncomfortable and drab and on the whole least thought is given to the patients' sitting-rooms. Chairs are very uncomfortable in rows along the walls or in front of the T.V. set. This lack of attention to day-room facilities is very much in keeping with the Americans disregard for sitting-room comfort in their own homes. Plans for improvements rarely concern the sitting-rooms.

Bathroom and toilet facilities seemed poor in comparison with the very high standards to which Americans are accustomed. There is no provision whatever for privacy. Even now toilets are being built in new hospitals without seats and with no doors at all. In some hospitals patients wash under cold running water at a communal wash-basin.

There are very excellent laboratories; clinical rooms; most elaborate arrangements for dentistry; chiropody; X-ray and every conceivable physical investigation and treatment. All hospitals have central supplies for sterile equipment and most have central linen rooms.

A very high percentage of beds is set aside for medical and surgical illnesses. I did not succeed in finding out why so many should be required but two possible explanations offer themselves:

Most hospitals would like to be accredited by the American Medical Association, by the Psychological Association, the Dental Association, etc., or they have just achieved accreditation. To do so there must be a wide range of experience available to resident students; and it seemed that this determined the provision for sick beds.

It is easier to obtain the services of physicians, surgeons, dentists, pathologists etc., than psychiatrists. Because the state hospitals have no link with other hospitals, they must employ their own specialists in every field, and must then find them enough work!

Most states allow more generous provision of nursing staff in the medical and surgical wards and it may be in the patients' interest to house as many as possible in these parts of the hospital.

The hospitals are generally divided into at least three areas:

Acute treatment wards. i.e. admission wards and acutely disturbed wards

Continued treatment wards. i.e. long stay wards

Medical and surgical wards.

Some hospitals have separate facilities for geriatric patients and for children.

All hospitals have good recreation rooms, many have bowling alleys, sports grounds. All have workshops and O.T. departments. All have canteens and shops.

Patient Care in Mental Hospitals

It is important to emphasise that nursing care is, in most instances, not given by nurses; but by people in other categories.

Nurses on the whole are not interested in psychiatric nursing. In the larger mental hospitals I have only seen nurses in the sick wards or in administrative or teaching posts. Some of the small wards attached to community clinics were staffed by nurses and in some of these the quality of care was excellent.

In most hospitals care is given by people who call themselves "Aides", "Attendants" or in California "Psychiatric Technicians". In some places attempts are made to train attendants as "Practical Nurses" or to employ "Licensed Vocational Nurses" in mental hospitals.

The terminology varies from state to state, so does the quality of care given. Some hospitals are able to recruit excellent people. Some gave a very good inservice training.

On the whole the patients are extremely well cared for, and I think we have much to learn from the American approach to inservice training. It was of interest to me, though, to observe that the comprehensive basic education which students receive is of no value whatever to the psychiatric patient. Nurses simply do not return to nurse and patients are in the hands of others, who receive a specialised training in the care of the mentally sick.

I was very favourably impressed by the general atmosphere in most of the hospitals I visited. Although doors are rarely open and it would probably be more difficult for American patients to leave hospital than it is for patients here, there was a tremendous feeling of freedom within the hospitals.

One hospital for the criminally insane, Atascadero in California, was an extreme example of how maximum security arrangements could be compatible with total freedom inside the hospital.

There is a noticeable absence of petty restrictions on patients. Routine is adapted to individuals, patients and staff are relaxed and relationships between staff and patients are cordial. In the grounds one sees large numbers of patients happily engaged in games or conversations, or going about their business. Even where patients are sitting about unoccupied, the feeling is relaxed, not apathetic.

This is, of course, not universal - there are some wards where patients are apathetic or where restrictive rules exist.

Morale is lowest, I thought, in the geriatric wards and in some of the children's wards, highest in the hospitals for the retarded and in acute treatment units.

Most mental hospitals are almost completely staffed with "aides, technicians or attendants". There are practically no domestic workers. Aides carry out domestic work and often some of the maintenance work in the hospital. They also act as drivers if patients have to be transferred or picked up from another hospital or even for taking visitors to the station.

There are some occupational therapists, some "rehabilitation workers", but the use of occupational therapy was not impressive. Quite frequently occupational therapists, like social workers and psychologists, function as psychotherapists.

There are "Volunteers" in most hospitals. Their function and usefulness varies greatly.

Food services are nearly always completely taken out of the hands of the nursing personnel. I have great doubts about the wisdom of this in psychiatry where food often has great significance to the patient. It may be that the giving and receiving of food is of less symbolic importance to Americans than to us.

Treatment

Psychiatric practice in the U.S.A. is much more influenced by psychoanalytic theory than it is in this country. Doctors have a long period of "residence" when they learn psychotherapy, but as far as I could ascertain, very little else. Physical treatment is strongly condemned at the moment as "old fashioned" and out-of-date. Drugs are used widely but not very scientifically as nursing observations on the effects of drugs are not available to the doctors.

Most doctors I have met are not really interested in hospital practice, they use it solely to become qualified for private treatment. It seems that hospital care suffers because so few doctors are interested in the life their patients lead when they are in hospital. Nursing care, consequently, is planned only in relation to individual patients, and not on the whole with a view to ward or hospital organisation.

In California there is a growing interest in the therapeutic use of the hospital environment and of the hospital community. It was most exciting to participate in the planning and discussion of the various schemes. Patient government, ward meetings of various kinds, patients' committees, patient organised newspapers, all aspects of what they call "Therapeutic Community" are being experimented with. The interest in this was awakened by a visit of Dr. Maxwell Jones and our concept of "Social Psychiatry" has great appeal. In the East on the other hand, the emphasis is very much more on psychotherapy and there is very little evidence that the role of the nursing staff has been thought out by the medical profession.

In all hospitals there are innumerable staff meetings - these are used more or less profitably in different places. Quite universally, nursing personnel are welcome to all case conference or team meetings and on the whole they participate well. I was surprised that as a visitor I should have had such free access to all conferences, many of which would have been very confidential in this country. At all staff conferences, clergymen of all denominations take part.

In many hospitals nursing staff did not wear uniform, in all of them the position of uniform was being discussed. It is widely believed that nurse-patient relationship is better if nursing staff do not wear distinctive clothing. Everyone is concerned about the fact that uniform tended to increase authoritarian attitudes. I was surprised that this was a problem to Americans, and I have remained unconvinced that the problem is solved by abandoning uniform, especially if the patients wear a kind of uniform in the shape of hospital clothing. It is good though to see nursing staff examining their attitudes so closely.

Some hospitals make very full use of ward clerks. Cardex system of record keeping is widely used. I was surprised that wards managed to find enough work for ward clerks and yet nursing staff were still busy writing.

Doctors give very detailed orders which appear to need endless transcribing. Often times I would have felt insulted had I been the nurse to receive such detailed orders.

Inservice Training

There is a widespread belief in the U.S.A. that training on the job is wrong, that it is educationally unsound and undesirable, and that it is only necessary because at the moment there are educational deficiencies to be remedied. Training is regarded with contempt as opposed to education which is greatly esteemed.

Having, observed the excellence of some of the inservice training and the poor standard of some of the education, I have become more enthusiastic than ever about training people while they are doing the work for which they are being trained.

In particular I became very excited about the first rate training given to the "Psychiatric Technician" trainees, in California. People of the very highest calibre are being recruited and within the first year are given 300 hours instruction before taking the Civil Service examination. The syllabus, the plans of instruction and the educational methods used, produce what I would call excellent "psychiatric nurses". Many hospitals take in new recruits every month and the training programmes in operation at anyone moment would put many nursing schools here and in the U.S.A.

to shame.

All hospitals have a "Director of Nursing Education". Sometimes she is responsible to the Director of Nursing, sometimes responsibility for service and education is strictly divided. It appears that one cannot say which of the two practices is to be preferred without taking into account the people involved.

In all cases the director of nursing education is responsible for the education of all nursing staff, not only the new technician trainees. At any one moment there is some kind of educational programme for every level of personnel. I was impressed the way new personnel were introduced to the hospital and with the universal interest in learning more about the job. It seems excellent that someone is specifically appointed to take an interest in the professional development of all.

If I were asked for the greatest single impression, I would stress the eagerness of all the technicians to learn more, and to keep informed of new ideas. Their willingness to try out new methods and to discuss with each other the progress they were making. This attitude, in my experience, is often confined to students in this country. That it perseveres seems to me due to the appointment on the staff, of a person whose business is education for all.

Nursing Organisation

I may have given the impression, until now, that all the exciting things in psychiatric care can take place without nurses being involved. This is my impression except that the "directors of nursing" and the "directors of nursing education" I met were, in fact, nurses of outstanding ability. So were the nurses in the State Departments responsible for nursing services in the mental hospitals. The U.S.A. is indeed fortunate in having nurses of such quality available for senior positions.

At the present moment, much as I should like to work in some of the State hospitals I have seen I would rather be a technician or aide than a nurse, as the work I find satisfying is performed by them.

In California, technicians are now licensed and the job carries full opportunity for promotion. Several of the assistants to the directors of nursing are technicians. In order to be eligible for promotion, technicians must take progressively more advanced examinations, and must show evidence of further study.

Technicians seemed to be well paid. Working conditions are good. A 40 hour week is universal and on the whole the technician can choose on which shift she wishes to work. Both male and female technicians work on male and female wards.

There is no equivalent position to that of our ward sister or charge nurse.

Although one technician occupies a charge position in the ward, this carries less responsibility and authority than the ward sister's post. There is less centralisation of information. The doctor retains more executive functions and there is always a supervisor for an area.

There is no hierarchy among the staff on the ward.

Although technicians have a great deal of satisfaction in their work, the position of technicians as a profession is, at the moment, uncertain. There is no recognition for them outside the state, even within California it may be difficult to find a job outside state service.

Nurses who are responsible for the success in creating the training scheme are uneasy in the professional relationships.

The Patient's Day

One of the most valuable experiences for me was to be in the ward, not in uniform, with nothing in particular to do, and to gain some insight into what life in a hospital is like. I was very much struck by the fact that even the best organised hospital life is meaningless for the patient. However full the programme, the patient's life consists of waiting. Waiting to see the doctor or waiting until someone makes some demand on her. It is difficult to see what motivation patients have to get up in the morning if the day has nothing to offer. Very frequently nursing staff had conceptualised very well how hospital life was meant to help the patient, but this was not experienced by the patient. It is my intention to see if patients here have a similar experience.

Nursing Education

Nursing education in the U.S.A. is sufficiently complex and controversial to cause difficulty in understanding, even among American nurses. Other people in the health profession are very ignorant of the nursing curriculum, and of the various grades of nurses. I was present at a staff meeting in one hospital when nursing education was explained to doctors, occupational therapists, social workers and others, who seemed very surprised at the situation.

It is possible to study nursing in a Diploma School, by taking a 3-year course in a hospital school of nursing.

There are college courses of 3, 4, or 5 years duration leading to a Bachelor Degree in Arts or Science.

There are 2-year courses at Junior Colleges, leading to Associate Arts Degree.

Nurses graduating from any of these courses are eligible to become Registered Nurses.

In addition there are Licenced Vocational Nurses, in some States called Practical Nurses, with a shorter education.

Diploma Courses and Degree Courses of nursing all follow comprehensive curricula, covering all the basic sciences required for nursing, including sociological and psychological subjects.

Clinical experience covers medical and surgical nursing, obstetrics, paediatrics, psychiatry and public health.

All schools of nursing are run as educational establishments with a teaching staff much larger than in our schools.

The students enrol in the school and are not members of the hospital staff. The school arranges their course, their timetable and their clinical experience and, wherever possible supervises their clinical practice.

Students pay for their education. In some diploma schools the hospital pays the student a small amount for their services in their senior year.

All courses I saw were very carefully planned. School brochures are most elaborate, very detailed, giving not only all the facts about the school, but also detailed course outlines. All schools have curriculum committees, enrolment committees, library committees etc. There is a lot of thought devoted to the development of the curriculum, to the logical progression of learning and to the integration of the various subjects. Students' health is well supervised, all schools have complete health services available. Counselling services for all students are considered to be of utmost importance and students get every help and assistance with personal problems as well as difficulties in studies.

All schools select their students with care, though the standard required for admission differs in different schools. All schools attempt to provide, in addition to a nursing education, a broad general education. There is great variation in the extent to which they succeed in their objective.

The aims of all basic nursing courses is to prepare the student for first level position in any branch of nursing. It is assumed that the student will later take advanced courses in specialised forms of nursing, and also in administration and teaching.

At the present moment there is strong disapproval among American nurses of Diploma Schools of Nursing. It is felt that some of these schools use the students for service and that the students' needs are subordinate to the needs of the patients. This sounded familiar to me, yet I must confess I saw no evidence of the students' needs being overlooked. In fact many of the diploma schools I visited appealed to me very much. In some of the Catholic schools, in particular, students seemed to have an attitude of enjoyment in giving service, which seemed most refreshing.

To understand the American disapproval however, one must see nursing education against the general educational climate which prevails.

It is the ambition of every parent to send the children to college and of every child to go to college. The whole nation is feverishly trying to solve the problem of how to provide enough schools, find enough teachers, and secure enough money for every school leaver to have a college education. Why this should be desirable was not at all clear to me, and it certainly seems an impossible undertaking in view of the tremendous growth of population. The desire to go to college is very closely linked with the idea of democracy and equality, at the same time it represents more even than material goods, the need for status and recognition. Few of the people I met are genuinely seeking knowledge for its own sake, the important thing is to "be well prepared" by having the necessary degrees.

A report of the State of New York recently published states that by 1970 80% of all school leavers will need college places. The report goes on to discuss how this can be achieved, but does not question at all whether this should be so.

Clearly if 80% of all school leavers go to college, colleges must provide courses in every kind of subject and must be the places where people prepare for their jobs. Most nurses must be recruited from among the 80% at college, and there is therefore no room for apprentice-type courses. It looks as if diploma courses will have to cease to exist. Two-year courses at Junior colleges and degree courses will provide two levels of preparation.

The 2-year courses seemed to me a very exciting new development. The students I spoke to were very determined to give bedside care and showed great understanding of the need for skilled nurses who chose to carry out practical nursing duties.

With so many schools of nursing in existence, it is obvious that there is very wide variation in quality of instruction. Competition for places in the best schools is tremendous. This is even more serious in graduate schools of nursing. In order to gain admission, students must show evidence of having attained very high marks in their previous studies.

Grades and examinations are terribly important to students. The anxiety about grades seemed to interfere with their ability to take full advantage of educational opportunities and the competitive spirit which prevails in schools of nursing inhibits cooperation among the members of the class. The necessity to do well in examinations also discourages students from trying anything really difficult.

Although courses are planned in great detail some students end up with surprisingly chaotic knowledge having obtained their degrees in part-time studies over many years and in different Universities. Every course entitles the student to a certain number of credits which can be collected in a quite haphazard manner. Many of the courses resembled evening institute courses or refresher courses of the kind organised by the R.C.N.

The advantage of schools of nursing being independent of the hospital and run as real educational establishments are tremendous. The students enter University with students in other departments. Many courses are shared, the social life, campus activities, clubs and academic interests of the University are available to nursing students. Standards expected from them are the same as for other students. Library facilities are excellent. The faculty is big enough to enable teachers to specialise.

Post-graduate students provide the necessary stimulus for advancement in the profession and research methods and attitudes are introduced early in the students learning.

Some of the teaching I saw was rather poor. This is partly due to the lack of well organised teaching courses. Partly it is inevitable, because of the very large numbers of teachers required.

Lectures and classes take place throughout the students' course. There is no block system or study day system. There are some classes every day, more in the beginning, fewer later, and sometimes classes are held in the hospital ward.

The clinical experience is planned to give the student progressive knowledge and understanding. This does not always work out in practice. For example, paediatrics is introduced early because it seems logical to learn about children first. Psychiatry comes late because the contact with mental illness appears to require a certain degree of maturity from the student. In fact, however, she may meet severely ill or dying children and very disturbed mothers in the early part of her experience which proves to be much more traumatic than the psychiatric problems she'll meet later.

Great care is taken that the practical learning is well supervised by clinical instructors and that repetition is avoided.

The result seems to be unsatisfactory. Students have very limited experience, lack self-confidence have far too few examples to fall back on when trying to apply theory.

I have become more convinced than ever that clinical instructors are not the solution to the problems of ward teaching. Students who have been instructed by clinical instructors only have never really observed nursing. I have discussed this with many students and asked them to describe to me good and bad nursing they have seen. They have not seen any nursing at all. They have only experienced their own efforts under the supervision of an instructor. They have no model at all, and, therefore, no aim for themselves. Worst of all they have never experienced the satisfaction of having been part of the ward team, of having been useful, of a job well done.

Much as I like the organisation of the classroom instruction and the planning of clinical experience, I should like the practical experience to be the responsibility of the ward sister. In psychiatric wards it seems particular inappropriate to have students for a few hours per day, if the students are in no way attached to the ward or involved in the life of the patients. Supervision by a clinical instructor can only be of use in this situation if the instructor spends enough time in the ward to become almost a member of the team.

Psychiatric Experience in the Comprehensive Course

There is some variation in the amount of time students spend with patients in different schools, and in the extent to which they take part in the events of the ward.

Theoretical work is extensive and it was surprising how much they managed to learn in so short a time. There is strong bias in all schools in the way psychiatry is presented and much of what is at best hypothetical is presented dogmatically as factual. Most schools are psychoanalytically orientated, even where the hospital has strong opposite bias. Some schools use Sullivanian theory. In San Francisco great emphasis is placed on "disturbed communication" in psychiatric illness.

Examinations are so constructed that the students are expected to classify information into 'right' and 'wrong', where this is totally inappropriate. Very few schools take the trouble to teach students to state their references or to know whose theory they are quoting. I found this surprising in view of the very careful annotation of text books. It was interesting to see the tremendous influence of Hildegard Peplau on all schools of nursing. Dr. Peplau's book *Interpersonal Relations in Nursing* is treated with the reverence only the Bible deserves.

The film *Nurse Patient Relationship* is shown everywhere. In the film a nurse helps a withdrawn patient by entering into a very special relationship with the patient. The effect the film has had on schools of nursing is tremendous. The special relationship - called everywhere a "ONE to ONE relationship" - is now considered to be the essence of psychiatric nursing and in many schools it is the only thing now being taught.

In the extreme form, the student is told that during her period in the psychiatric ward her sole duty lies in finding a patient with whom to form a relationship.

The student is left to make her own choice, find her own way of approach and decide for herself how often to see the patient, in what circumstances and what to do with her.

At least weekly the student discusses with her instructor, in detail, the inter-relation between herself and her patient, special attention being paid throughout to the student's feelings. The student learns to recognise her own feelings of anger at being rejected, pleasure of being liked, need to be popular, fear of failure etc. She understands how her feelings influence the patient, how feelings find expression, how she can deal with her own emotion. She prepares carefully for separation from the patient.

I was impressed with the skill of some instructors in helping students to examine themselves. These instructors state, quite frankly, that the only purpose of the psychiatric affiliation lies in providing the student with a pause during which she learns about herself.

This is thought to be valuable in helping the student to grow and mature. I think if it is well supervised, it also helps her to understand the mechanics of emotional involvement and gives her skill in entering into involvement without harm to herself.

I was completely unable to find out how this is supposed to benefit the patient. Indeed I found no reference in all this to what was happening to patients while a succession of students formed relationships with them. At no time did I hear the relationships discussed specifically in connection with the patients' needs or difficulties. No student or faculty member was able to tell me what specific benefit they expected a patient to gain, and what special forms of relationships seemed indicated by the patient's condition.

The patients themselves and the psychotherapists seemed blissfully unaware of the impact of this relationship which the student thought to be so important.

I do not feel entirely critical of the "one to one relationship". It seemed a useful way to ensure that emotional involvement is taught and not left to chance. In this country we sometimes either believe that involvement should be discouraged, in which case the student feels guilty when she does become involved, but receives no help. Or we encourage involvement, without, however, proper safeguards for the nurse. American nurses are aware of the problems created by involvement and try to deal with them.

I do not think, however, that this is the only thing that should be taught and I am left wondering about its relevance to psychiatric nursing or to nursing in general.

At the end of her experience, the American student is in no way equipped to function in a psychiatric hospital. I am not convinced that she is better equipped to nurse elsewhere because of the psychiatric experience she has had, but I am assured this is so.

The instructors concerned with teaching students during the psychiatric experience hold themselves responsible for changing students' attitudes, for promoting sympathetic understanding of patients, for personal development and for creating sensitivity to social and psychological difficulties. They also invariably feel they must teach the students about growth and development before they can begin to teach psychiatry.

It was surprising to see that the gulf between psychiatry and the rest of nursing is as great in the U.S.A. as it is here, and that after years of inclusion of psychiatry in the curriculum there is allegedly still so little understanding of psychological problems among those who work in surgery or medicine.

Advanced Studies, Master Degree Programmes, Doctorate

The purpose of the basic comprehensive course is to prepare the student for first level positions in nursing. All specialisation and advanced knowledge is meant to be taught in master degree programmes.

I enrolled at Boston University as a special student, to participate in such a programme. It would be totally misleading to compare this with advanced degree study in this country. Rather one should think of the master degree as the equivalent to a post certificate course. My colleagues in the master programme were wholly ignorant of psychiatric nursing. In 18 months they were to learn some theory of psychiatry, psychology and related subjects, and they spent approximately 8 hours per week in clinical experience in the hospital. Of this about 4 hours per week were to be spent in a one-to-one relationship with a patient. A little experience in conducting group discussions was also included and a short piece of research work was to be carried out. The students with a master degree in psychiatric nursing are then considered specialists. Some of them later work in psychiatric wards, but most of them find teaching posts in University schools of nursing.

The result is that psychiatric nursing is being taught by people who have never done it and the patients are being cared for either by totally unprepared nurses or by aides.

In the few wards where I saw really first rate psychiatric nursing, the people concerned told me that they had acquired their knowledge by trial and error and by conference / discussions in the ward in which they were working. Their course had not prepared them, except in the most general sort of way, by giving them the background education. Some master programmes have a slightly broader base, but the general trend is the same.

Because nursing is taught in universities and most schools of nursing have attempted to become full university departments it is necessary to have a university faculty which is as well qualified as in other departments.

All university departments have at least some professors who hold doctorates and consequently there is great pressure in nursing to find some people capable of taking higher degrees. Courses are only just developing and everybody is aware of the difficulty in finding suitable content.

Research is an important aspect of advanced work. There is certainly no shortage of suitable candidates for the courses, if and when they are developed.

Research

I took part in many seminars on research methods in nursing, and paid particular attention to any research projects in which nurses were involved.

The fact that at all levels, nurses are taught to investigate nursing problems is most exciting. Instead of being expected to do things the way they were always done, just because they were always done that way, nurses are taught to plan research projects and to submit everything they see to critical examination and evaluation. It was astonishing how accepting hospitals are of students who come into the ward to carry out research.

The actual quality of the research seemed on the whole rather poor. Much of what is called research really does not deserve the name. In the long run, however, valuable findings can only be made if people are prepared to look. The quantity of research and the general enthusiasm for it should bear fruit in the future.

Male Nurses

There is a shortage of male nurses in the U.S.A. Most schools of nursing do not take male students. Some schools will accept male students, but have very few. The only schools which have a sizeable number of male students are schools situated in mental hospitals. I saw three of these, two in New York State and McLean Hospital in Boston. These schools appeared very good to me, but are not looked upon with favour in the U.S.A.

Canada

I spent much too short a time in Canada to form any opinion of the Canadian psychiatric hospitals or nursing education in Canada.

The few days spent at Montreal and Toronto were most stimulating and I enjoyed the very high level of discussion which took place and the excellent teaching I was able to observe.

I am deeply grateful to Miss McColl for the tremendous trouble she has taken in making arrangements for my visit. The time spent in the offices of the Canadian Nursing Association and in the offices of the Nurses Association in Toronto was greatly appreciated.

I was particularly glad to have the opportunity of meeting Miss Helen K. Mussallem who had recently completed a report called "Spotlight on Nursing Education". Miss Mussallem had directed a pilot project for the evaluation of Schools of Nursing in Canada.

The report she has written is one of the most interesting documents I have ever read. Many of its findings are relevant to nursing education in this country, and the criteria used for evaluating schools of nursing merit special notice. Detailed study of the report is strongly recommended.

Conclusions

Many of the impressions of the last year are still waiting to be sorted and properly digested. I saw many excellent examples of teaching and nursing which will need to be thought about before some of what I learnt can be applied.

Three main points have mainly occupied my thoughts:

The general pressure to adopt comprehensive training worries me all the more, now I have seen it in operation in the U.S.A. It is not at all clear what precisely psychiatric experience can contribute. Attention to the students' own development should be possible in any ward and at any time of her training. Knowledge about patients' emotional problems can be gained at any time. Special knowledge about psychiatrically ill patients cannot be gained in a short time. Psychiatry tends to attract people who may not generally be interested in nursing and who would be lost to the profession if the separate register is given up. The psychiatric patient certainly does not gain from this. I found the manner in which students were introduced to psychiatric wards most disturbing. Large numbers of students coming together, leaving within a few weeks disrupt the ward. I do not see how this could be avoided in this country if all students were to have psychiatric experience.

I became tremendously interested in the training of other nursing personnel. The scheme for technicians in California in particular would serve as an excellent model for training of psychiatric personnel. At the moment it is relevant to our planning for enrolment. Should the mental register be closed we might have to think along the same lines as the United States in training people who are not nurses to do the job. Inservice training for all staff was of great interest.

While I was not entirely impressed with nursing education in the U.S.A., I was very envious of the ability to attract very highly intelligent people into nursing. It seems that the fact that nursing is studied at a University makes this possible. There seems to be less discouragement of the brightest in the U.S.A. In the schools of nursing the brightest students receive all the encouragement and stimulation they need to do well and progress rapidly. Parents and schoolteachers seem less prone to dissuade the brightest pupils from entering nursing. In the hospital they have scope for their ability and enquiry is encouraged. Whatever the shortcomings of nursing are in the U.S.A. at present, there seem to be enough first rate people in nursing to remedy these in the future. It seems while we may be rightly proud of present standards of bedside nursing in this country, our system does not encourage future leaders to enter nursing now. Some way must be found to recruit and retain at least some of the university type of student into nursing without losing our advantages of training.

Paper 3

Report on visits to state hospitals in California in June, July, and August 1960

A. Altschul

First of all, I should like to express my sincere thanks to Dr. Blain for enabling me to visit the hospitals, clinics, and other facilities of the Department of Mental Hygiene.

My most outstanding impression throughout my stay in California is that of the hospitality, kindness and helpfulness of people everywhere, in the office at Sacramento, and wherever I went. It is impossible to thank individually all the many people I was fortunate to meet. My special gratitude however is to the Superintendents of Nursing and their assistants. I am deeply conscious that without their cooperation, and indeed their welcome, my visits would have resulted in dismal failure. I have reason to be indebted to them and to many other members of the nursing personnel for much personal help and guidance. I should like to thank them for the hard work they have put into the preparation for my visits and during my stay.

My particular thanks also to Mrs. Steele, Mrs. McClelland, and Mr. Thrailkill whose help and encouragement was beyond measure.

Although I am here concerned only with the official part of my program I feel that what little understanding of problems I have gained and whatever awareness I have, of special characteristic of American or California society, is in large measure due to unofficial part of my tour and to the wonderful people I now proudly call my friends.

Most of the comments I wish to make here, have already been made during staff conference in August. I should like however to summarize the main points.

In the course of the three months I have visited the following places:

1. Hospitals for the mentally ill:

   Atascadero
   Camarillo
   DeWitt
   Mendocino
   Metropolitan
   Napa

2. Hospitals for the retarded:

   Fairview
   Pacific
   Porterville
   Sonoma

3. Langley Porter Clinic

4. San Joaquin (Short Doyle programs)

   San Mateo

Gereral Observations

With the exception of Camarillo Hospital, where I spent 3 weeks, I spent 2 or 3 days at each of the hospitals. Each one had planned my stay differently and it was interesting to observe what use was made of my time.

Everywhere I was shown some wards or departments. Naturally the time available for this varied as did the selection of what I was shown. I should like to emphasise that any opinions I have formed are based on the very incomplete sample of the work I was shown. In some hospitals I was shown the best, in others I was shown those areas about which the hospital was most concerned; in some hospitals I had difficulty in discovering whether people were pleased or displeased with the particular aspects of work they were showing me.

In some hospitals I was asked to address large groups of staff, usually of multi-disciplinary nature. More often I met with small groups of people. Sometimes these were convened according to grade in the nursing structure, e.g., groups of nurses separately from technicians, or assistant superintendents separately from charge nurses. At other times I met with groups of people working together in one unit or one ward. Frequently I joined in meetings which would normally have taken place anyhow, e.g. team meetings or clinical conferences. In some hospitals I was invited to attend patients' meetings, and on several occasions to address patient groups.

In retrospect I feel I gained most from being allowed to see the hospital working normally, and from meetings with small groups. I am well aware of the degree of security and the level of morale required to allow a complete stranger to participate in discussion of internal problems and I am deeply appreciative of the opportunity offered to me. Wherever I was able to meet patients and move freely among them, it was possible to gain some idea of staff-patient relationships.

Although I now express a preference for informal meetings with small groups. I would not have liked to influence the arrangement made in any way.

I was greatly impressed by the variety of facilities available, of method of treatment, of standards of care, and of special emphasis of interests, both between hospitals and within the same hospital. There appeared to be unlimited scope for initiative and ideas. Sometimes I felt that personnel were unaware of this. Some of the frustrations complained of by some people did not seem to exist for others. Some of the outstanding examples of individual initiative did not appear to be perceived as such by the people concerned.

Among nursing personnel, nearly everywhere, I was struck by the enthusiasm, desire for progress and change, capacity and willingness to discuss, and the loyalty to their hospitals.

General Topics of Discussion

Among topics most frequently raised, apart from questions about England, were problems related to Ward Management, Therapeutic Community and Patient Government.

My impression was that ideas on these were hazy. It was taken for granted that these were good things but nursing personnel had not attempted to define the concepts, examine the rationale, or view these ideas in relation to other forms of treatment.

In some hospitals medical policy with regard to these ideas had been put into operation with totally inadequate preparation of nursing personnel. Nursing personnel are left with a tremendous sense of responsibility for ward management, which they feel has passed out of their control. They do not realize how much scope they have in a therapeutic community and feel fearful of expressing any opinion. They are resentful when their traditional role is criticized. There is a great deal of misunderstanding of concepts like "democratic ward management". In their anxiety not to appear authoritarian many have simple abdicated from responsibility for making decisions. At the same time they feel, rightly or wrongly, that doctors, relatives, and "the public" will blame them if anything goes wrong.

The concentration of interest on ward and hospital management, group approach to therapy and group activity, results, in my opinion, in lack of knowledge of individual patients.

Some form of summary of case histories should I think be provided to nursing personnel, and it should be part of their function to report about individual patients behavior, attitude, and progress. The specific aim in treatment as it affects individual patients has been lost sight of, no less, in many cases, the goal of discharge to a specific set of circumstances.

Some problems appeared pressing in only some of the hospitals.

Among these were the care of geriatric patients, use of restraint, problems related to children, to alcoholics, to physically disabled. Some of these will be referred to under later headings.

Buildings and Physical Environment

The sight of brand new hospitals was very strange to me as there has been practically no building program in England. I could therefore not help but wonder to what extent planning had taken place to facilitate nursing and aid recovery. I must confess I did not find out.

The advantage of large wards totally escapes me, even assuming they were more economical to run. The large space caused fatigue or feelings of helplessness and an institutional outlook among personnel. There is constant reference to "so many patients" one does not know what to do! There is a tendency to distribute jobs among personnel rather than divide up the patients into small groups. Nobody gets to know the patients. No patient can develop any relationship with a particular employee. Space is utilised for mass movement. All patients eat at the same time, over-crowding the dining room leaving the rest of the ward empty, or they are all in the sitting room, or all in dormitories, or all in washrooms. I do not see this as the most economical use of space, or as a preparation for normal living. It would seem possible to me to nurse the patients as if the wards were divided into smaller units, but all the people I spoke to told me it was impossible.

I wondered why it was thought desirable or necessary to have toilets without doors; or total lack of privacy in the shower rooms.

My most serious objection to large wards concerns the old people. The physical exertion for old people making their way from bed to chair or chair to toilet is tremendous. Incontinence is increased through force of circumstances. When patients become helpless, the nurses' work of getting patients out of bed into chairs is made much more heavy by distance.

In order to arrest confusion in old people and help them to orientate themselves, their living space must be made simple and have some clear landmarks. Personal property must be clearly distinguishable and bed, chair, and clothes must be recognisable. This is not the case in large dormitories, where all counterpanes are alike, or in large day rooms with chairs in rows, all identical in pattern. It may be possible for the aged to remember a few faces, but not hundreds. The resulting loneliness is pathetic.

While I feel that my dislike for large wards may be irrational in other respects, I am certain that large wards are detrimental to the care of the aged.

Furniture, Ward Layout and Catering

I have seen many wards in which nursing personnel have used initiative and ingenuity to make the atmosphere homey. There are many personal touches. In some wards chairs are so arranged that patients can converse, display of personal property, handmade ornaments and provision of drapes have made many wards pleasing. On the other hand, in many wards chairs are arranged in rows, there is total lack of embellishments and patients never speak to each other.

Restraint is widely used to protect patients from falling off chairs or out of bed. (I have seen little restraint used for other reasons.) I am certain that most restraint could be abolished if more attention were paid to the suitability of chairs and beds for the patients who use them. There should be upright chairs to facilitate rising, and low ones, or rocking chairs to prevent getting out. Variety of pattern of chairs is necessary when there are people of different build, different ages and different deformities.

I would put acquisition of suitable, safe, adaptable wheelchairs very high on the list of priority if patients are not to become prematurely bedridden.

Eating Arrangements

Eating arrangements in wards where patients are helpless are not always satisfactory. Many patients precariously balance their trays on their knees and eat in solitude in the wards.

I was struck by the difference in approach to these problems in different hospitals. It is my impression that the hospitals for the retarded have been much more successful in obtaining and devising suitable chairs, tables, and walking aids for the disabled, than have the geriatric wards in mental hospitals.

Relationship between Public and Hospital

Nursing personnel are extremely conscious of their patients' difficulties on discharge. They believe that the public are unenlightened. They feel in some way responsible for protecting the hospital from the public and adopt an attitude of defensiveness to visitors, which may be instrumental in alienating them. Some of the rules about visiting, the notices addressed to visitors, appear to indicate that visitors are not welcome.

Nursing personnel are afraid of criticism from visitors and are unable to make the best use of patients' clothing or property because they will not risk any damage.

While the nursing staff are acutely aware of their responsibility in fostering good public relations, they have difficulty at times in accepting internal hospital policy which they feel might increase the risk of public criticism. In particular they are afraid of giving patients freedom of movement for fear of accidents, afraid of encouraging mixing of sexes for fear of moral indignation, afraid of open doors for fear of security risks. There is a great need to clarify the purpose of the open door policy. It often means an aimless wandering of patients in the grounds instead of inside the ward. Personnel are often not aware that the open door requires of them greater vigilance. Not less, but more purposive activity, better observation and more personnel.

The degree to which nursing personnel can be held responsible in the event of incidents, needs to be clarified.

Occupational Therapy

I was struck by the absence of material for Occupational Therapy. True, many patients work on "industrial" assignments of more or less therapeutic nature; however, the more sick patients have nothing to do. It has always been my understanding that a full occupational program is a *sine qua non* of a therapeutic community, or of a policy of open doors.

What is the purpose of tranquilizers if there is no alternative to inactivity and boredom? I do not know how one assesses the effect of drugs if one has no occupation for patients.

I have seen many individual attempts made by nursing personnel to provide patients with useful activity and raise patients' self esteem. Often personnel have taken along their own materials and given them to patients. Some useful examples of training patients could also be quoted.

Any more effective use of occupational therapy would, however, require:

- a clarification of the roles of rehabilitation and nursing personnel.

- a clear financial policy.

I was frequently told that there is no money available for materials, e.g., for dressmaking or embroidery. On the other hand, I was told that it was against the rules to sell the finished product to raise money.

It seems that if material is to be provided free, it needs generous budgeting. The more successful occupational therapy...the more material needed. On the other hand, probably the less money needs to be spent on drugs.

However it might be possible to make occupational therapy almost self-supporting, if reasonable prices are charged for finished work. Many articles now purchased could well be made by patients, e.g.. clothing. Much work in the hospital could be therapeutic for patients, as furniture repair, painting. Emphasis on the value of group work projects and on the socializing effect of work, on the usefulness and value to the community could make work projects truly therapeutic and minimize danger of cheap labor.

I mention this because it is so important for nursing personnel to know what the policy about work is. They know that it is bad for patients to sit about. They feel guilty, yet there is nothing to help them in what I consider to be one of the most important nursing functions - motivating patients for work and creating in them the social skills which come with work.

If however I am mistaken, and it is the current belief that work is not important then this should be made clear to nursing personnel to free them from their sense of guilt when patients are idle.

Definition of Roles

Not only in relation to occupational therapy, but in many other activities, the nursing functions overlaps with that of other people. I know this is inevitable in teamwork, however, there are situations in which this appears harmful to the patients. What for example is expected of nurses with regard to entertainment?

If the rehab department initiates entertainment but is not there to see it through, cooperation of nursing personnel is essential to success. Very often they display a lack of interest, because nobody has explained to them the value of the specific program. Patients become discouraged owing to personnel attitudes.

The greatest need in clarification of roles seems to exist in the children's departments of the mental hospitals where teachers, psychologists, occupational therapists, play therapists, psychiatrists, social workers, volunteers and nurses all appear to carry out similar activities. There is no evidence that nursing personnel understand the over-all policy or know their own function. In all this the children, appear to me to lack continuous normal home life and background, and there does not appear to be anyone who helps them to grow up and develop an aim and direction in life, while hundreds of people concern themselves with their treatment.

In contrast, a very clear and purposive approach prevails in the juvenile boys ward (Ward 13) of Camarillo and in most of the wards for the retarded children.

Definition of roles also seems to me desirable in relation to group therapy. I was told of this being practiced by psychiatrists, psychologists, social workers, "group leaders", nurses and technicians.

If group psychotherapy is practiced, skill and knowledge is required which nursing personnel do not have. If something else is meant, I have been unable to get an explanation.

I am aware of the need of patients to belong to a small group and can think of many ways in which nursing personnel can help patients with such identification, but I have not found any nurse who could explain to me what her aim, her technique and her achievements were.

I was repeatedly told of the value of teamwork and the need for understanding among personnel. This does not to me appear to preclude a division of labor, or a definition of the special contribution each worker can make.

Volunteers

I was impressed with the magnitude of volunteer programs, but wondered if the volunteers would not obtain greater satisfaction if they could adopt specific patients for visiting or to give presents to. I did not quite understand their motivation, or all their contributions.

Selection and Training of Nursing Personnel

I found this aspect of my experience of particular interest. My over-all impression is that of wholehearted admiration for the quality of nursing personnel. I was tremendously impressed with the calibre of both nurses and technicians in senior position, and by the very high quality of recruits the hospitals are able to attract.

At top level I was quite unable to distinguish between nurses and technicians without being told. The intelligence and aptitude of many of the trainees would be the envy of every nursing school in England.

The favorable impression I have formed of the technicians raises in my mind a whole lot of doubts, which I am sure have been resolved already in the minds of those concerned. Why for example try to attract nurses into the field at all, when technicians do such splendid work? Is the work of technicians different from nursing, and their training more appropriate?

The fact that technicians can be promoted to senior positions lends support to the belief in equal status. But the fact that they can only be promoted in certain wards leads to distortion in status, not only of personnel, but also of patients. I find it difficult to understand how one encourages a belief in the worth-whileness of the technician, and at the same time suggests that something is to be gained by taking up a nursing course. Is, on completion, a junior nursing appointment to be preferred to a senior technician?

I find it hard to see how the nurses engaged in teaching trainees reconcile their work with their own professional interest. If they succeed in producing good technicians where does nursing stand! If they have no interest in furthering the professional status of technicians, how can they do a good job in teaching?

I know that in many hospitals these problems do not exist. In some hospitals however, there is a certain amount of friction. I had never thought of myself as excessively professionally-minded and in many ways I am surprised that these should be problems to bother me when they obviously don't worry the people concerned.

I am full of admiration and envy of a system in which every worker has some in-service training.

I was unable to discover what determines the curriculum and on what grounds decisions were made.

There was frequent reference to the examination at the end of the course. No one seems to know what it consists of and whether it is in fact relevant. Some hospitals, the examination in mind, teach things they themselves do not consider important.

Examination results are good and this is referred to with pride.

I do not understand this view of examinations. If most people pass it seems to indicate either that the exam is too easy or that the students received excessive instruction. There is little to show the relationship between teaching and examination, or to indicate the validity of the examination in determining suitability for the job.

It would be interesting to know what would be taught, were it not for the exam. Is the aim to prepare the technician for work in his own hospital, or in all hospitals? Retarded as well as mentally ill? Atascadero as well as other hospitals? Private institutions as well as state hospitals?

Methods of teaching depend largely on the number of trainees which have to be taken in. As this is dependent on many social factors beyond the hospitals' control, it seemed that the numbers of trainees bore no relationship to size of hospital. The number of nurses engaged in teaching, however, is determined by number of beds. For this I can see no justification.

All hospitals would like to be able to carry out clinical instruction, but clearly this is impossible in some hospitals due to lack of teaching staff. There is wide difference of interpretation of 300 hours teaching. In some hospitals this is all given in the classroom, in others it includes clinical instruction.

Student Nurses

I have not had much opportunity to observe content and method of student education during their affiliation. Different schools appear to have different ideas, even where they use the same hospital as "laboratory". I find this term quite repulsive and cannot believe that one can acquire appropriate professional attitudes if one looks upon patients as laboratory material.

I am not clear how the students' experience during affiliation fits in with the treatment the patients are having, or with any work the student will later be required to do. I am particularly dubious about much of the psychoanalytic terminology and its relevance to the treatment of patients. It was frequently explained to me that American psychiatry is dynamically orientated, presumably meaning based on psychoanalytic theory. There is however no evidence of this in the day-to-day management of patients.

I shall have opportunity later to observe training through one to one relationship. My observations so far leave me dubious of its value.

Short Doyle Programs

I found the visits to the two community hospitals extremely interesting. The answer to problems with the public, to education of the community, relationships with general hospitals and to overcoming the difficulties created by large hospitals, may well lie in the development of community clinics. At San Joaquin I was particularly impressed with the educational and public relation efforts. At San Mateo I was stunned by the volume of work and the excellent quality of psychiatric nursing.

I would like to conclude by referring again to the many examples of superb work I have seen in every hospital and by paying tribute to a system which attracts so many outstanding people, encourages them, and maintains their morale.

I have in this report concentrated on difficulties because I believe nurses can benefit most, for themselves and for the patients, if some of their problems are brought to the attention of people.

The fact that such excellent work is done in spite of difficulties, and that in most hospitals I experienced profound concern and feeling for patients speaks for itself.

Once again I should like to thank all the people I have met for their help, and Dr. Blain for giving my tour his blessing.

Paper 4

Evaluation of one term at Boston University School of Nursing

A. Altschul

This evaluation must start with an apology for the long delay before its production and dispatch. When I left in December 1960 I had every intention of writing down what I thought and felt before allowing too much change to take place. However, I became involved in new experiences so rapidly and intensely that it became impossible to devote time to this report

Perhaps it is best that I should now look back upon the three months at Boston in the light of all subsequent experience and with feelings tempered by the passage of time. Possibly a more realistic appraisal is now possible than might have been at the time of departure.

I should like to take this opportunity to thank the Dean for accepting me as a student; Miss Mellardi for her interest and help throughout my stay; Miss Godbout for the tremendous trouble she has taken in arranging my programme, and following my progress; and all members of the faculty for giving me so generously of their time. Above all I should like to thank them all for their friendship, kindness and hospitality, and all their many personal contributions to the fullness of my experience.

I should like here, to anticipate what should perhaps be the summing up of this report, and stress again how much I appreciate the personal interest people have taken in me. My memories of Boston University will remain permanently influenced by the personal relationships I have enjoyed.

Having observed other students receiving similar treatment from the faculty I feel that one of the greatest assets of the school lies in this personal relationship between faculty and students. What I have admired beyond all else is the flexibility of a nursing school, which enables each student to follow his own curriculum and to have individual supervision, counselling and advice.

I shall presently try to assess the value of the semester's work in relation to each course I followed. Before I think specifically of these I must, however, refer to the total picture. As I write this I am conscious of my difficulties in recalling my initial aims. I gained so much from my stay which I could never have anticipated or planned that I no longer feel my aims have any relevance to my experiences. The multitude and diversity of learning experiences I found available to me went far beyond anything I could have envisaged and many of the satisfactions are unrelated to the original purpose of my enrolment and possibly to the intentions of the university.

I believe I have gained some knowledge about nursing education, in at least one notable School of Nursing. The fact that I remained longer at Boston than at any other place in the U.S.A., that I made friends, had colleagues and met people from varied walks of life, helped me to gain a little insight into some aspects of life in the U.S.A.

Having visited several other schools of nursing, both collegiate and diploma, after leaving Boston University, I have been able to compare since, nursing education of different kinds. My contacts with nurses at all levels in many states have helped me to see nursing problems in the U.S.A. from within, rather than with reference to my own preoccupations. At Boston University I was sufficiently involved to see nursing problems from the point of view of the student, the faculty, the staff nurses of the hospitals I visited, the medical profession and the public.

I was unable, however, to set aside, even for a short period, my rather firm conviction that nursing is a service to the community, and that students of nursing should learn to serve and to nurse.

This attitude of mine has frequently led to my being accused of being "Service Oriented". I gather that this is one of the worst insults of which American nurses are capable. I can see the advantages of full student status, without however being wholly convinced that education and service need be as far removed from each other as I felt them to be at times.

When I referred to the total experience I included the value of having had enough spare time to be interested in things outside Boston University - books, newspapers, radio, television, shows and films characteristic of the American way of life. I also visited several hospitals, was in touch with State Departments of Mental Hygiene in Massachussetts and Connecticut, with Public Health Departments, and with other universities. I counted among my friends a number of doctors, I met people who had children at school and who viewed nursing from the point of view of the parent.

I met people who had been nursed. Discussion with all these provided a healthy counterbalance to the collegiate opinions.

Most valuable of all was, I think, the opportunity of having colleagues and of belonging, of sharing with other students their aspirations, satisfactions, disappointments and criticisms. Everywhere else during my stay in the U.S.A. I was only a visitor.

I would not have missed the experience of living in Franklin Square House for anything. Few visitors to the U.S.A., I am sure, have the opportunity of submerging in the ordinary life of the community, the way a resident at Franklin Square House does. Not only in relation to nursing but in every respect, for example, during the fascinating months of the election campaign this was an education in itself.

I should like to comment on each course I attended.

Biostatistics

Having taken statistics before, I had no great difficulty in following the course. I found the course quite outstanding. The subject was made crystal clear without oversimplification. Its application to the biological sciences became comprehensible to me for the first time. I enjoyed statistics without having to worry about arithmetic. The method of presentation was interesting. I enjoyed the lecturer's general approach and appreciated the fact that he treated the class as adults. This latter remark might imply that I found this approach unusual enough to emphasise it. At the time this is the way it struck me. In retrospect however, I find that all the members of the faculty were prepared to treat students as grown-up. Somehow the students insisted on behaving like school children. This lecturer resisted this very firmly and made the class aware of its attitude.

Dr. Apple

This course was to me a source of pure enjoyment. As I only audited this class I looked upon it as an example of first rate teaching demonstration, and spent all my time observing Dr. Apple's method.

Her manner of utilising every contribution from the class no matter how trivial, irrelevant or inaccurate, was a delight. I was fascinated by the way she pursued her line of development giving the appearance of allowing the class to determine the direction. I marvelled at her way of summarising and of extracting the essential facts from the mass of material offered by the class. I would have described Dr. Apple's teaching as representing my concept of perfection. Having enjoyed the course more than I can say, I was surprised how little some of my colleagues had leamt from it or appreciated it. In this course, more than in any other, I became aware of my fellow students desire for formal, didactic teaching. On meeting students in their 3rd semester, I was amazed that they were ignorant of facts I knew Dr. Apple to have taught.

The value of this course lies perhaps in the stimulus it has provided for a critical re-analysis of my assumptions about educational methods.

Miss Mellow - Theoretical Basis of Psychosis

In this course I found it difficult to adjust to my role as a student. In many ways I felt more like an observer noting the tremendous variation in knowledge and background of the students, and Miss Mellow's skilful way of adapting her teaching. From time to time I had trouble with the role of an outsider.

When I felt most detached and complacently superior to some of the students and identified with the teacher, I contributed nothing. When I participated more actively, I felt guilty about monopolising the class. It seems to me that my presence must have been somewhat disruptive and detrimental to the other students.

It was of great value to me, to think very seriously about the way psychoanalytic concepts can best be taught. I started on a train of thought which I shall pursue for some time to come, namely to determine what really are the theoretical foundations on which psychiatric nursing is based.

I cannot accept the belief that Freudian psychology is the only, or indeed the most important theoretical framework. Even if it were, I have so far failed to see where in psychiatric nursing it is applied. I have however nothing to put in its place, having for many years managed to practice and to teach psychiatric nursing without troubling about theoretic foundations. The search for foundations impresses me. The uncritical acceptance of a hypothetical theory as factual, does not.

At some stage in this course I developed an interest in Existentialism. Whether this was an incidental or deliberate by-product I do not know. I am glad I was not concerned with "grade averages", as my preoccupation with this fascinating and to me new philosophy, prevented proper concentration on assignments. I wonder if my American colleagues are wise in allowing grades to become so important in their lives. How much of the potential benefit of a university do they miss if assignments. worry about examinations and grades, limit their interests.

It was a source of great surprise to me to find that some of the master students knew practically nothing about Psychiatry. This set my thoughts wondering about the effectiveness of the basic preparation, and the place of the psychiatric experience in a comprehensive basic course.

I was also surprised that few of my colleagues appeared willing to defend their opinions if they were challenged, or seemed to enjoy pursuing an argument. This may have been due to their courtesy to me as a stranger, or they may have interpreted my enquiries as critical and may have reacted defensively.

Dr. Standish's Group

I greatly value the privilege of participating in a group of this kind and of being allowed to join in its last semester.

I felt a full member of the group very rapidly and gained a great deal. I was interested to observe Dr. Standish as a leader on the rare occasions when I was sufficiently detached.

I am not sure whether I made sufficient use of the group to learn theoretical concepts from its own dynamics, or whether any of us could apply knowledge gained from it in any future situation in which we may find ourselves in the capacity of group leader.

Miss Weymouth and Miss Scott's Seminar

This was probably the most useful course in a straightforward, direct way. It was part of my aim to see what research was going on in psychiatric nursing and to learn something about research methods.

The course fully satisfied me, though I am aware I did not satisfy the instructors.

It would have served no purpose to have completed a rather poor piece of research in the short time available. I benefited from planning and from the criticism of the plan. Of course the weekly exercise of examining other people's plan was of great value and the brilliance of Miss Scott's grasp and analysis, a constant object for admiration and envy.

I am grateful for the discipline of the methodological approach to research. In retrospect I am not sure that the results justify the means. Most of the research reports I read appear to deal with trivialities. I could not help feeling that the process of researching and publishing mattered more than knowing about the subject matter.

Of course it is clear that only a scientific approach can lead to improved nursing practice and that some nurses must leam to look at nursing with a researching kind of eye.

I was very impressed with the willingness of nurses to be researched upon and the generally enquiring attitude which results from the emphasis on research.

Field Study

This should probably be assessed under a number of different headings, of which I shall only mention three.

1. The opportunity of seeing at least one hospital from the point of the student, and incidentally the patient and the staff, was invaluable. Enough has been said elsewhere of my impressions of the hospital. My main concern as a student was with the therapeutic relationships with my patient: I could not fail to observe, however, the quality of nursing, the inservice teaching and the education of students from various schools, which was going on around me. I cannot come to any conclusion about the students, and don't know if there should be some relationship between the performance of the qualified nurse and the effectiveness of student education. My reluctant, though only tentative conclusion, is that there must be something wrong in a system of education if the end product is poor.

2. The fact that I had much time to mingle with patients, to be in the ward without being busy and without responsibility, also that I was allowed to attend morning reports and clinical rounds, has helped me to look more closely at the patients' life in hospital. I cannot easily accept that patients should waste so much time just being in hospital without making hospital life in itself therapeutic. Nor can I believe that the sole function of nurses is to form relationships. Relationships are important, providing they are specific to the patient's need, are established in the course of business arising from the patient's daily life, and are used by nurse and patient in the shared life in the ward. What I observed was the students' attempt at establishing relationships without any apparent purpose and out of all context to the patient's treatment in the ward. I was interested to note the importance students attach to the relationship, the total disregard of these relationships by all other members of staff, and the patients' unawareness of the significance. The patients' utilisation of the hospital day will be my subject for study for some time. The experience of working in an entirely psycho-analytically orientated clinic was new and stimulating.

3. The experience of working with one patient in a one-to-one relationship.

It would require more detail than I am able to give here to assess this part of the course. My personal changes and adjustments would have to be discussed.

Miss Mellow and I were, I think, both aware of my resistance to involvement. I worked through a good deal of personal difficulty without making all of it explicit. The regular skilled supervision, I received, was nonetheless the essential part of this experience, enabling me to deal with the formation and dissolution of a multiplicity of relationships. At the same time I was also trying to observe what effect this kind of teaching has on the patients concerned, and to learn how I could use what I experienced in my future teaching. I would have liked to be able to compare what was happening to me, with what I could discover about the experience of my colleagues.

Spreading my interest so widely may not have been a very good idea as it may have strengthened my resistance and delayed involvement.

At this stage I view the experience as satisfying and valuable. This method of teaching helps the student to understand and cope with emotional involvement. Providing each student is as fortunate as I was in having experienced supervision, it is an excellent practice. When I think of some of the graduate students I met at Boston University and elsewhere, and visualize the supervision they will be able to give, I shudder.

Though I concede that there is value in this to the student, I have remained entirely unconvinced of the value of relationship therapy or nursing therapy, to the patient - in fact it seems patently unfair that students should use patients to leam about their own psychopathology. Perhaps one should recommend a personal analysis for all nursing students. Interpersonal relationships between patients and students should have some validation beyond the satisfaction this gives to the nurse.

It is easy to counter all these objections by pointing to the fact that I remained detached and used defences against greater emotional involvement. Had I experienced more fully the impact of involvement I might have become more convinced of its value. This kind of argument would render nursing therapy as invulnerable and as immune to criticism as psychoanalysis is already. If only the initiated and the converted are entitled to discuss, and only to praise not to criticise, one cannot wonder at onlookers who dismiss the subject as unscientific. As a partial onlooker I remain doubtful.

I should like to include in this evaluation my thanks to Mrs. Hargreaves for discussing with me the problems involved in teaching undergraduate students and for helping me to understand nursing education in the U.S.A. In spite of all her efforts I did not quite succeed in understanding the American educational system, or the place of nursing education within it. This fault lies partly, I think, in my limited perspective at the time, partly in the "insularity" of Boston University and of Boston itself.

Throughout my stay I was conscious of local colour influencing my thinking. Not until I left did I become aware of the extent of this influence. It seems perfectly possible to complete one's studies at Boston University without ever realising that other people, other places, are doing interesting work, both inside the U.S.A. and beyond. The predominance of local references in bibliographies was one aspect of this which struck me forcefully. The more subtle implications escaped me until after I had left Boston.

The bias towards degree courses in nursing was obvious and understandable - in a collegiate school. I did not investigate how valid were the criticisms of diploma school or what were the sociological influences on the nursing profession of the U.S.A. These are topics I have been thinking about since leaving Boston University.

One of the results of my ignorance at the time was that I could not properly compare the School of Nursing with anything else. However, one can not keep learning new things entirely without comparisons.

If I compare the education of the Boston University student with that of student nurses in Great Britain, I find the Boston University student has tremendous advantages. She has a well planned curriculum, and learning experience, full student status, all the facilities of an educational establishment at her disposal. She has the stimulus of a campus environment, the library, the laboratory facilities of a college, good vacations, no responsibility. She is expected to think primarily of herself.

People who enter nursing in Great Britain and in the U.S.A. are very similar I think. On the whole British School leavers are as well educated as American ones, even if they leave earlier and have fewer paper qualifications. The bulk of recruits come from a very similar range of ability and intelligence. However, it is my impression that the really brilliant student in the USA has more encouragement, less opposition and prejudice to overcome than her counterpart in the United Kingdom: The American nursing profession should find it easier than the British one to find its highly gifted leaders and teachers.

The average newly qualified nurse in Great Britain is on the whole quite as knowledgeable as her American counterpart, in spite of less theoretical teaching. She has so much more practical experience that she can deal with theory much more rapidly.

Those who complete their training in Great Britain are, I feel, no worse than American nurses. Many students however, in Great Britain, do not complete their training. I understand that Boston University has no great problem with attrition. It may well be that Boston offers the student more satisfaction than British Hospital training does.

It is pointless to compare Boston University School of Nursing with university life in Great Britain. The present level of university selection is so high that most nursing students would not have a chance at all.

There is a very different approach to teaching in Universities in Great Britain whether they use tutorial or lecture methods. There is evidence that some British universities are widening their sphere of influence. Future developments may well follow American trends. The inevitable reduction in standards if the percentage of admissions rises would be a disadvantage in many respects though nurses may stand to gain.

If it is difficult to compare undergraduate studies at universities, it is impossible to compare post-graduate studies. The term "post-basic" used by World Health Organisation, would seem to me more apt for the specialisation courses I have seen at Master level at Boston University. The Diploma of Nursing or the Sister Tutors Diploma correspond in Great Britain with American Masters degrees. What precisely is involved in a Doctorate in the U.S.A. I did not find out, and my colleagues appeared as baffled as I was.

I ended the semester at Boston University full of admiration for the best which is achieved, and for the personal qualities and erudition of the faculty.

I ended, disappointed with the mediocrity of some of the students and I am left puzzling how the system of education in which I was so generously allowed to participate produces such widely dissimilar end products.

Paper 5

Report on the One-to-One Relationship with Mrs X, Boston

A. Altschul

Mrs X

I have been seeing Mrs X four times a week since the beginning of October. During most of the time, meetings took place in the ward, and on each of these occasions I spent only approximately one to one and one-half hour with Mrs X, but one-half day in the ward. This was deliberate, as I wanted Mrs X to perceive me as a nurse interested and concerned with nursing matters. I also showed interest in other patients though emphasising that my visits were specially planned with Mrs X. During recent weeks there were several occasions when we went out together and three visits to the Xs' home.

I made it clear to Mrs X that I was a nurse and unable to give her psychotherapy. She had difficulty in understanding what kind of help I was offering, and to some extent this was my fault, as in the beginning I was none too clear of my own role. There were many occasions when Mrs X tried to force me into a psychotherapeutic role and much evidence of her resentment of what she considered second-rate therapy. She has very definite ideas of the nature of "therapy" and repeatedly impressed upon me that I could not hope to understand her without hearing all about her past. During the first few weeks, she tried to set the stage for psychotherapy by lying down on her bed as soon as I arrived, inviting me to sit in a low armchair beside her bed.

Mrs X gave me many detailed accounts of the short-comings of the various members of her family. I consistently expressed interest, but on every occasion returned to the problem Mrs X herself has in dealing with the situation. I used such comments as: "I can see how difficult this must be for you. How can I help you to manage better (with your children or husband or household)?" Or, "It is impossible for me to change your husband. I should like to try to help you with your difficulty."

Relationship with Mrs. X

It is difficult for me to assess what the relationship with me has come to mean to Mrs X. She became very anxious about wasting time whenever a silence occurred, or whenever she felt she was not telling me what I wanted to know. I tried to convey to her that there can be some value in simply being together, enjoying companionship, liking each other. I sympathised with her very real difficulties and tried to convey to her my belief in her personal worth and trust in her ability to be successful. Periodically, this has been difficult because Mrs X repeatedly puts herself in the worst possible light, almost forcing me to become disapproving. However, I think she has begun to develop some feeling for me. Once or twice she has demonstrated a little tenderness; on one occasion she appeared relaxed and gay. A few times she showed emotion in her depressed state and indicated her desire for support from me. The most frequent show of feeling for me was a sudden burst of anger or loss of temper. She suggested the use of Christian names.

We discussed many times Mrs X's difficulty to give and receive love and friendship. Her relationship with husband, children, mother-in-law, friends and myself were discussed. When Mrs X talks about feelings, there is usually very little evidence of it. Her feelings are demonstrated in her action. There is a repetitive pattern of inviting love, and then repelling it at the crucial moment; of giving feeling, and in the last moment spoiling it by sudden bursts of hostility. In my visits to Mrs X's home I saw this pattern of behaviour towards family. At the hospital, she demonstrated some of it in her approach to other patients and her dealings with personnel. Mrs X's difficulty in accepting and giving is at times expressed in her attitude to presents or offers of cigarettes. She does not believe in the sincerity of the giver, and she feels that she should never give except in precise measure of return. The problems of giving and receiving were acted out between us and discussed when Mrs X gave me a bracelet she had made in the day hospital, and accepted from me fertiliser for her plant and a pamphlet about dogs.

Problems Discussed

Her difficult relationships with husband and children came up repeatedly. Without fail, Mrs X began by describing the family's shortcomings, often doing it in such a way that her own method of antagonising them was obvious. I frequently led her to look at her own attitudes, but this she has only done by the use of verbal cliche, not with any emotion. It is obviously too difficult for her to look at herself. She blocks completely and says she cannot remember, or talks of her guilt feelings without any evidence of feeling at all.

She sees the situation of housing, social position, money and the problems of her husband's deception and her children's emotional disturbance as completely hopeless. She refers to her children's problems as it she were talking of case material, without any involvement.

I have tried to find out how she visualises success, and what she feels she would be like if she were well. Her concept of success is causing me some difficulty. I have never met her type of materialistic outlook. There is a totally unrealistic ambition of social advancement. She values material possessions for their own sake and professes interest in middle-class cultural values such as music, of which, however, she has no knowledge. She approves of the philosophies of a competitive and acquisitive society, and has a profound contempt for work. Her own and her husband's failure cause her feeling of hopelessness and resentment. She wants to own money and beautiful things but does not wish to use her possessions. She can not see the point in giving the children toys, as they might only break them; or to paint the furniture while the children might again draw on the paint. She does not see herself in any way active in bringing about change. Her husband owes it to her to provide. She can only contemplate change if her husband finds a better job or a second job or becomes more efficient. She herself does not feel she should do anything at all towards improving the situation.

We discussed at length the problems with the children. As I see it, her greatest difficulty lies in her total inability to give feelings at all to the boys. Y, the older boy, comes to her at times, but she instantly rejects him. The little one does not come near her. She did not discuss her feelings for the children at all. Responsibility for them is seen by her to consist in physical care and creating discipline. We spent a lot of time talking about the children's development and going into detailed observations about their play, their speech, their behaviour. Mrs X does not know her children at all and passes the responsibility for their treatment off to various agencies.

Problems of running the household were also dealt with by discussion; and on home visits, by attempting to deal with them. Again, I tried to go into details against a good deal of resistance.

At the moment Mrs X feels trapped. She does not think she is improving and feels that the hospital will not keep her forever. Rather than be transferred to the State hospital she would like to discharge herself. Whenever she contemplates doing this, her anxiety increases. She feels she might as well be home, yet she knows she can not go home. Her panic at night makes it impossible for her to leave the hospital. I have not found any way to get her to discuss her feelings of fear. When anything approaches the topic of sex, she immediately stops talking altogether.

Since a patient in the yard successfully committed suicide, Mrs X has not spoken of killing herself; before that, she mentioned it occasionally. She would like enough medication to overcome her depression and anxiety. The problem of medication has frequently been raised by her. I have felt happier when Mrs X was sufficiently anxious to be motivated to look at her problems. Increased sedation causes her to relax and exploit being sick to the full. On the other hand, I have been worried about her depression and agitation on a number of occasions. She attributes extreme agitation to pre-menstrual states.

I think some progress has been made in focusing on Mrs X's own difficulties instead of talking of the husband's shortcomings. She has been weaned to some extent from the use of psychoanalytic jargon, but I suspect this is only temporary, to please me. The main difficulties arise from Mrs X's inability to pursue emotional topics. She blocks or changes the subject, and with me found it easy to draw red herrings. It is not yet clear just how far she is ready to allow change to take place in herself. My feeling is that she has too much investment in being sick to risk changing.

In spite of my attempts never to give my own opinion or to influence Mrs X's action, she has taken action with a view to pleasing me. Her present frequent visits home and her purchase of a dog appear related to her interpretation of my views.

Mrs X's age is given in the documents but is not included here to ensure her anonymity.

7 December 1960

Paper 6

Feedback to Supervisor, June Mellow, on One-to-One Relationship with Mrs X

A. Altschul

It is never easy to sum up impressions, experiences, and events. After a period, so rich and varied in learning situations as my last three months, it is almost impossible. My attempts at recapturing what was important or in highlighting what was noteworthy result in producing a kaleidoscopic effect of images, memories, and ideas, in which nothing remains stable long enough to allow for adjustment of focus and develop precision of definition. Perhaps, at the risk of being called a cynic, I could express what I learned at Massachusetts Mental Health Center thusly:

Never, under any circumstances, allow anything at all to be published. Always strive to remain in complete obscurity.

Any hospital following these prescriptions for success would find itself short of students and visitors. This would have the advantage that permanent personnel would find time to think about patients. They would receive some recognition and consequently gain some satisfaction from their work. It would also give the hospital the advantage that people like me would be spared the disillusionment I experienced and would not feel so critical and dissatisfied.

As I attempted to sort out my ideas and put them on paper, I found myself becoming increasingly critical. All the hospital's and personnel's shortcomings were listed, not a single favorable comment would come into my mind. Obviously, such wholesale condemnation must find its explanation in the eyes of the perceiver. No place could possibly be as bad as the Massachusetts Mental Health Center of my description. I tried to find what caused me to be so dissatisfied. However hard I looked I could not detect in myself any signs of depression, which might have accounted for my selection of facts. My gloom is restricted to the way I think about the one hospital. In all other respects I am able to find enjoyment. My own past experience is not responsible for setting my expectations irrationally high. On the contrary I am very conscious of throwing stones from a glass house, Eventually, I think I discovered the reason for my dissatisfaction which led me to formulate the new philosophy I stated earlier. I am angry because the hospital is not the way its own publications make it out to be. My expectations were created by the writings which have come out of the Mass. Mental Health Center. The hospital itself had created an image of itself which renders reality unrecognisable.

When I realized what was wrong I went back to the book which had served as my Bible for years - From Custodial to Therapeutic Care in Mental Hospitals. Sure enough, one by one my criticisms of the hospital turned out to refer to failure to come up to its own standards. True, there is no longer any emphasis on custodial care, there is now no care at all. True, there is no physical restraint, it is unnecessary because the hospital will not treat disturbed patients. There is nothing in the book which would lead one to expect the amount of sedation and the volume of tranquillizing medication used in lieu of understanding. Therapeutic atmosphere and environment was not in my inspection restricted to furniture. I did not expect the state of total confusion in relationships to which patients are exposed. Perusal of the book led me to expect a high standard of professional education. I found nursing personnel as ignorant as or more so than in other hospitals. Nothing in the book prepared me for the atmosphere of dislike of patients, disapproval of sickness, and absence of sympathy! I expected frequent communication between the various disciplines - I found meetings for report which were simply an exchange of ignorance and an opportunity for creating ill feelings. No other staff meetings, no attempt to deal with problems of patients or staff by group discussion, no exchange of information about individual patients.

Little regimentation in the ward, it is true - instead there is total disinterest in patients' activities. The value of activity, specifically applied to individual patients is discussed in the book. In reality patients are permanently idle and bored without even the incentive to get out of bed or attend to personal appearance. The few young, active patients who can not control their behavior when there is nothing for them to do are punished by being restricted to their room, still with nothing to do.

There is much in the book about the value of democratic attitudes. I failed to detect any sign of it in the ward. Anarchy, chaos resulting from disinterest in patients, and vindictive use of personal authority when the patient forces attention.

I am becoming bitter again. Certainly my feelings are out of proportion to the situation. Perhaps my involvement, in trying to work with a patient, was great enough to fan the flames of my indignation. Most of it, however, was there even before I had found a patient.

In all this I am strongly reminded of a book I read a long time ago. Arthur Koestler in *The God That Failed* describes feelings which apply to me. His disillusionment with communism was certainly of more importance than my disillusionment with M.M.H.C. His ability to describe and explain feelings is a much better way than mine and I shall end referring the reader to Arthur Koestler hoping here to spare me an occasional thought and to remember that big feelings can apply to little problems.

References

Greenblatt M., York R. H. & Brown E. L. (1955) *From Custodial to Therapeutic Care in Mental Hospitals*, New York: Russell Sage.

Commentary 1

Reflecting on times past ...

Annie Altschul

At the time I applied for a scholarship of the Commonwealth Fund for Nurses, the General Nursing Council for England and Wales was encouraging schools of nursing to develop 'experimental schemes of training'.

We had made a contract with three schools: Kings College Hospital, Hammersmith Hospital and St. Bartholomew's Hospital, to accept students who had volunteered to spend two or three months of their General Training on a psychiatric placement.

I had no idea at all what to try to teach them during this secondment All my experience was with two or three year courses and my approach to gaining knowledge about psychiatric patients was rather leisurely.

I don't think I had formulated my aims very clearly at the time, but in retrospect I would put them this way: Since both patients and students spent a long time with each other, the first priority was to make the students comfortable and to help the student to become accepting and non judgemental.

Since patients were admitted to hospital because they had difficulties adapting to the demands of society, the business of the ward was to adapt to the patients. What the hospital had on offer to the patients was the opportunity to learn better adaptive modes of behaviour, with respect to the routines of living, with respect to forming relationships with people, both male and female, people of all ages, people over whom they had authority and people who had authority over them. Perhaps because my early psychiatric experience was in a military setting, I accepted the belief that all patients had to have a job, because only then could one judge whether the patient was capable of coping with work related stresses.

All of this seemed to me the function of the interdisciplinary staff team. But I was particularly influenced, I think, by the research I had read about Chestnut Lodge in the USA, where patients seemed to receive an hour's psychotherapy each day, but where the question was asked of what happened to the remaining 23 hours. These hours seemed to be regarded as the responsibilty of the nursing staff. If these hours could not be used therapeutically, then the patient should perhaps not have been there at all.

I believed that only a small amount of the nurses' time, and only with a few of the patients, would be spent in a one-to-one relationship, in what might have been seen as a competitive relationship with the psychotherapist, or at times, perhaps as a complementary relationship. I thought of this aspect of psychiatric nursing as the most difficult part of the job and one which the student could only learn at a late stage of training, at a time when she felt secure in her other functions. I had, however, been profoundly influenced by Peplau's work with withdrawn schizophrenic patients, as illustrated in the film *Nurse-Patient Relationship*, and I had become aware of the apparently mutual avoidance of relationships, as described by Gwen Tudor Wills, and I wondered how the student nurses who were only to have a brief encounter with psychiatric patients were going to cope with these situations.

After considerable consultations, I was advised that Boston University might be a useful place to visit in connection with my search for meaningful short experience for student nurses, and when I was awarded a Fellowship I applied there and was offered a place as a 'Special Student', i.e. I was simultaneously to study the experiences of young student nurses, of their supervisors and of the Faculty members concerned with the teaching during psychiatric placements.

To my amazement, when I was awarded the Fellowship my hospital offered me a full year's leave. Three hundred and fifty pounds was clearly not enough to survive for a year. The State Department of Mental Health for California offered me the opportunity to run a series of workshops for their 'Psychiatric Technicians', which I took up before I went to Boston. Thus I saw the effect on permanent staff of student nurses' one to one work in psychiatric wards, before I had the opportunity of studying the benefits of this experience for students and for patients.

On return to the Bethlem Royal and Maudsley Hospitals, I made much use of the newly found knowledge, but I remained unconvinced that it fitted in naturally in the psychiatric scene as I found it in the U.K.

By the time I came to Edinburgh, the 'Wider Basic Training' for all student nurses had been introduced. Students in the new Degree course in the University were just starting their psychiatric experience, so it followed quite naturally to develop my interest in the topic in what was for me a new and welcoming setting.

Commentary 2

Annie Altschul: An American Perspective on her Commonwealth Fund Visit, 40 years later

Shirley A. Smoyak

Professor Shirley A. Smoyak, RN, PhD, FAAN; Professor II, Rutgers University, the Bloustein School of Planning and Public Policy, 33 Livingston Ave., New Brunswick, NJ 09801

In 1960, when Annie Altschul visited the United States, Canada and Australia as a Commonwealth Fellow, she was in mid-career. I was just beginning my own, having finished a Master's degree with Hildegard E. Peplau as my mentor. While I have met and talked with Annie Altschul over the years. I am very sorry that I did not get to meet with her and have professional discussions about psychiatric nursing during her American visit. What a shame! So many of the comments that Annie has made in the 50 pages of summary and evaluation shared with us by Steve Tilley could have been the beginning of a wonderful dialogue. I am almost to the point of grief about this missed opportunity. It may sound a bit bold, but I truly believe that psychiatric nursing in both the United Kingdom and the United States could have been dramatically positively influenced had such a dialogue taken place.

Why Annie's itinerary was constructed as it was remains a mystery to me. There's not a clue regarding why she did not visit Hildegard E. Peplau and the innovative graduate program at Rutgers University, which emphasized clinical practice rather than administration or education. That focus was totally new at the time and quite controversial. It's clear from her Report to the Commonwealth Fund that she knew of Hilda's work and also knew that she was regarded as a powerful figure in the profession. Quoting from her report: "It was interesting to see the tremendous influence of Hildegard Peplau on all schools of nursing. Dr. Peplau's book, *Interpersonal Relations in Nursing* is treated with the reverence only the Bible deserves."

The two talked many times over the years, mostly in conferences held in the United Kingdom. I do not know whether or not Annie ever shared this perspective with Hilda.

I will organize my comments by the degree to which I see Annie's statements (from within all the documents we had for review) as being particularly profound, insightful, important, forward-looking or disturbing. Annie has a wonderful way of making short, brusque, to-the-point statements which often are very far from the reality seen by others. She often says things that others might know, but are embarrassed to admit. Some of her comments are so directly and boldly stated, that she might as well have shouted them. It is a pity that she rarely gives an example of some point she has made, nor does she provide any documentation. My comments and rejoinders, then, are couched as comparatives from my own experience and the literature. We cannot argue her points without having clinical data, actual interviews or statements by patients and staff, course syllabi and the like to which she had access during her visit. Nevertheless, I think that all of us can learn from her and from each other's viewpoints during this conference. I will arrange my points according to my judgment of their importance or value. Each point will be labeled as a paraphrase from Annie's work.

Point 1: Psychiatric technicians or aides do more actual nursing than nurses do

In the United Kingdom, there is no such level of personnel, and Annie found their existence in the United States to be intriguing. Apparently her visits within the California State system provided the most opportunity to learn about their training and how they delivered care to state hospital patients.

Annie tells us that her intent had been to learn about how psychiatric nursing was integrated into comprehensive nursing training. To her, "training" is a suitable word, and one which describes the process of learning on the job, or within the wards, with senior nurses as role models. The apprentice model is one that is a comfortable one for her and her colleagues. She sees "education", particularly education occurring in a university setting as aloof, too divorced from the real word, and loaded with unnecessary ideas and facts. She thought it was totally silly that so many Americans aspired to having a college education, even if only at the junior college level. For her, a college education probably does not ensure learning to be a nurse because direct experience is missing.

But technicians work on the job and learn directly how to do the tasks that are necessary. Their training is "real" not theoretical and lofty. Here's the important point that Annie misses. Technician or aide training is task oriented. Technicians deal with things to do, not ideas. They ensure that patients are well fed and well dressed. Why they have landed in a psychiatric hospital is not their concern. Technicians do not know how to administer medications, nor do they know which side effects are most dangerous. They do know how to take temperatures and blood pressures, but cannot act on their findings.

Annie enthusiastically describes her California visits. "In particular I became very excited about the first rate training given to the 'Psychiatric Technician' trainees in California. People of the very highest calibre are being recruited and within the first year are given 300 hours instruction before taking the Civil Service examination." The most amazing sentence to me comes next. "The syllabus, the plans of instruction and the educational methods used produce what I would call excellent 'psychiatric nurses'". (My emphasis). To me, this statement produces a huge bewilderment. How could a woman who is such an excellent observer, has such a fine mind, and can deliver wonderfully articulate policy analyses say such a thing? My effort to understand how she could see rigor and quality in such brief, atheoretical teaching or training methods challenges my brain. Personally, I want to fly with a pilot who understands wind velocity effects, aerodynamics and physics, not just one who learned to fly by sitting next to other pilots who say, "Do this and that".

Maybe what Annie observed in the technician training was a

comfortable cognitive match with what she had observed in the UK. Mental nurses are trained separately from the general nurses, and are not required to understand, in depth, anatomy and physiology or biochemistry. Their focus is on mental processes and not how the body works. The UK mental nurses probably know more about communities than most American RNs. Of course, having both the technician syllabi and the syllabi from the UK mental nurse training for comparison would answer that question.

Furthermore, I am convinced that the aides' level of expertise in the American East is far different from the West, even in the '60s. The aides or technicians in the East are barely high school graduates. Their command of language is generally poor, and they take positions in state hospitals because they have no orientation to work as a career. It's just a job. Even our auto mechanics are more serious about their commitment to their work.

I have never seen Annie conduct an interview with a patient, or provide hands-on psychiatric care, so I cannot tell what it is about the technician that fascinates her. For me, they have largely interfered with my teaching on wards with both graduate and undergraduate students. They do not want new ideas introduced into what they perceive as "their" domains. They want patients to just sit and do as they are told, not be active and engaged in any therapeutic process. Ironically, Hilda and I presented summer workshops at Napa State Hospital in California, where Annie visited. The aides would deliberately see to it that the most violent, unreachable patients were selected for us to do the work of teaching how to do one-to-one dialogues, or engage in the nurse-patient relationship described by Hilda. When we managed to do the teaching without being hit or punched, the aides were amazed.

Point 2: Nurses on the whole are not interested in psychiatric nursing

This is another amazing statement. With so many other choices to make, why would a nurse select a field she or he does not like?

Our education has mental health nursing as just one of the fields for which undergraduates are prepared and they can select among many clinical options.

Further, for 20 years, Hilda and I conducted summer workshops across the United States for nurses in state hospitals who wanted to learn new and better ways to help psychiatric patients. The workshops included foci on both individual and group processes. Some included material on how to conduct studies in ward settings. These began in the late '50s, and were in operation during Annie's visit.

Annie does not mention the National Institute for Mental Health, which was first funded in 1946. This government body awarded individual grants to nurses to continue their education, and also awarded schools who wanted to develop clinically oriented Master's curricula.

Psychiatric nurses in the late '50s and '60s published more than nurses in any other specialty, and they were the first to organize certification processes. If that's not interest, what is it?

Point 3: Psychiatric nursing needs no theoretical basis and is not psychotherapy

This view of Annie Altschul's departs dramatically from what American nurses believe. Annie states that she has not been burdened by having to justify what she is doing with some theory, so I would love to have a long conversation with her about how she decides to do and say what she does when she is working with patients. At the same time that she is saying that she does not need theory to practice, she presses others to tell her how they define psychiatric nursing. In an article in the *Journal of Psychosocial Nursing and Mental Health Services* in 1984, with Annie Hargreaves as the interviewer, Annie Altschul made many statements that sounded exactly like her evaluation materials from 1960-1961.

Annie apparently thinks Freudian psychoanalytic approaches

are useless, and I would agree that this is the case with severely psychotic people who cannot cooperate with the talking process. But to discount as useless all of what psychoanalysis has to offer puzzles me. Furthermore, there are theories that are quite useful in working with people who are very, very disturbed. Harry Stack Sullivan, for instance, worked with patients who were diagnosed schizophrenic. Peplau studied with him at Chestnut Lodge, and used his ideas in her own work and with her students.

I cannot understand why Annie went along with June Mellow's admonition to not do psychotherapy. In fact, 31-year-old Mrs. X, who was visited by Annie for months, did engage in a psychotherapeutic relationship with Annie, although Annie would protest that she had not done this. Digesting the 5-page summary, dated the 7th December 1960, can only bring the reader to the conclusion that this was psychotherapy. Annie invited Mrs. X to see her situation in alternative ways, and asked her to consider the outcomes of her actions. There is no doubt that Annie was trying to get Mrs. X to have a new perspective and to try new lenses.

Annie also tells us that she had no particular goals when she engaged in study at Boston University. With no goals, then how do you know when you've arrived? I suppose that it is possible to take a trip or even a long journey without an itinerary or a set destination. To me, however, that would be quite unsettling. I need to be grounded by at least having an area or a country in mind.

Point 4: Nurses cannot describe what they do, or what psychiatric nursing is

Annie seems to take issue with the popularity of the one-to-one relationship as a teaching tool. She may have seen some inappropriate teaching, where the faculty focuses more on the students' feelings and experiences than on the nurse becoming competent to help patients to see how their life events have shaped outcomes.

From my earliest days of working with psychiatric patients I was able to explain what I do. In a nutshell, I helped patients to understand their current situation as an outcome of what they had learned and experienced in the past. Sometimes medications did aid the process of recall and analysis. I like to point out, however, that I was a psychiatric nurse before Thorazine (chlorpromazine). The efforts were to develop strategies to make changes in how things were understood and/or interpreted. New actions were planned and implemented. These included knowledge of managing stress, managing relatives and managing medications. The focus was always on the patient, not the nurse.

Group work was used to explore living together in community settings. Resolving disputes, sharing strategies for interpersonal communications and relationships, and airing different points of view were all appropriate foci.

Some examples of how she asked the question, and what the nurses answered, would have been helpful.

Point 5: Money is spent on the wrong things

In describing the paucity of materials for occupational therapy, and the unattractive day rooms or open areas on wards, Annie laments that the policy makers need to think more carefully about how they allocate fiscal resources. In her view, too much is spent on drugs, and not enough on materials for occupational therapy projects.

She also points out the stupidity of having a policy that states that patients cannot sell what they make in occupational therapy. Obviously, this would provide a source of funds for new materials.

As a related point, she observes that most nurses do not understand the funding processes, and are unaware of how money is allocated for the various areas and projects within hospitals. Nurses also are rather fuzzy about what or who dictates how the work will be done among team members. For instance, she shares observations of nurses being unwilling to continue what a recreational therapist has begun.

Point 6: Boundary issues between professions and staff affect patient care negatively

Unfortunately, Annie does not give us any actual descriptions of a dispute or a battle over turf, but what she says does resonate with me. Social workers who do not worry about community resources or discharge plans, but instead engage in talking with patients, appear to be indistinguishable from psychologists or psychiatrists. Annie is amazed that nurses do not object when physicians or psychiatrists write very detailed, demeaning notes, demanding that regimes be carried out. She could not understand why they did not see this as an insult to their professional capacity. I agree wholeheartedly.

Point 7: Hospital structures are planned poorly

Annie saw many new psychiatric facilities being built, a very different phenomenon from the old structures in the UK. However, she wondered how the planning had been done because space utilization was so problematic. She could not see the advantage of large wards, housing 60 or more patients, or hospitals with thousands of beds. Even if the answer would lie in the area of economy– just easier to run than small units– large space causes fatigue and a feeling of helplessness. An institutional look does not feel like home.

In a very astute observation, she shares her distress that space is utilized for mass movement. "All patients eat at the same time, overcrowding the dining room while leaving the rest of the ward empty, or they are all in the sitting room, or all in dormitories, or all in washrooms. I do not see this as the most economical use of space, or as a preparation for normal living." Well said.

I cannot help but comment that the technicians are in charge of those arrangements, in many instances operating the units as if they were military barracks.

She also is bothered by the fact that toilets do not have doors for privacy, even in the newly built facilities. Poorly designed furniture for older patients is also a concern. Chairs and beds, which have the potential to create falls, need to be re-thought. More wheelchairs are needed. Her view was that restraints were used to prevent falls, and that the better approach would be to have more comfortable and safe places to sit and rest.

Another design feature that was poorly thought through were the lack of landmarks for older patients with poor eyesight. Disorientation is more frequent if one room or bed or chair looks just like all the others. She eloquently ends that section with "The resulting loneliness is pathetic."

Point 8: Research is talked about, but not done

Annie tells us that she paid particular attention to nursing research, particularly in the psychiatric field, but saw none. There were some stellar examples of psychiatric nursing research, dating back to the '50s. I cannot fathom why some of these were not pointed out. For instance, Gwen Tudor (Will) (1952) studied mutual withdrawal on a psychiatric ward. She showed that patients would use gestures or actions that were disturbing or provocative, and then repeatedly used these when they discovered that so doing would produce an avoidance by the nurse. Her study report included examples of verbatim exchanges.

Hildegard Peplau prepared an historical analysis of trends in psychiatric nursing, which was known as *The Williamsburg Report* and until published in A Collection of Classics in Psychiatric Nursing Literature was shared as a purple ditto. While not an experimental design, it certainly was historical research. *The American Journal of Nursing* printed Peplau's first work on loneliness in 1955. That article showed how case data could be used to construct and test theory.

In early continuing education workshops, ward studies were a part of the curriculum. When Annie visited, most undergraduate programs did not have a research component, but most master's level programs did. She is correct, however, that there were few published studies.

Point 9: Public health nurses and psychiatric nurses are collaborating with each other

Altschul astutely notes the very beginning of a trend– that Public Health Nurses were becoming increasingly concerned with their role in psychiatric work, and were even studying psychiatric nursing in post-graduate courses. They were among the first to use research projects in order to attempt to identify the best nursing strategies at different points in the illness continuum. She also notes that Public Health Nurses sought out their colleagues in psychiatric nursing to provide nurse-to-nurse consultation.

What's not mentioned:

1. The different roles that UK nurses play with forensic patients, when the security function is combined with the nursing function. In the U.S. they are separate.

2. How the Commonwealth Fund used her reports.

3. Whether fuller versions of her observations and analyses were ever done.

4. Whether these 50 pages have been generally available to the nursing community and others.

5. Whether she ever had any response from June Mellow about her work with Mrs. X.

References

Hargreaves, Annie (1984) Interview with Annie Altschul: Psychiatric Nursing in Great Britain, *Journal of Psychosocial Nursing and Mental Health Services*, 22, (1), pp35-40.

Peplau, Hildegard, (1956) "Historical Development of Psychiatric Nursing: A Preliminary Statement of Some Facts and Trends," in Smoyak, S. and Rouslin, S, (1982) *A Collection of Classics in Psychiatric Nursing Literature Thorofare*, NJ: Slack, Inc.

Peplau, Hildegard, "Loneliness" *American Journal of Nursing* 55, December 1955, reprinted in Smoyak, S. and Rouslin, S, (1982) *A Collection of Classics in Psychiatric Nursing Literature Thorofare*, NJ: Slack, Inc.

Tudor, Gwen E. (1952) "A Sociopsychiatric Nursing Approach to Intervention in a Problem of Mutual Withdrawal on a Mental Hospital Ward" *Journal of Interpersonal Processes*, reprinted in Smoyak, S. and Rouslin, S, (1982) *A Collection of Classics in Psychiatric Nursing Literature Thorofare*, NJ: Slack, Inc.

Commentary 3

'Returning to Whence I Came' – based on conversations with Annie Altschul

Peter Nolan

Professor Peter Nolan, School of Health, Staffordshire University, Blackheath Lane, Stafford, ST18 0AD

Introduction

I first heard of Annie Altschul shortly after I commenced psychiatric nurse training in the early 1960s at Tooting Bec Hospital in South London. Three of our tutors, Una Budge, Pat Barry and Derek Godderham would frequently refer to her in their lectures and it was obvious that she was a person who commanded respect among psychiatric nurse tutors. Una was particularly eager to impress on us just how much Annie had achieved - the speed with which she had mastered spoken and written English, the extent of her travels, the quality of her publications and the work she had done to establish a theoretical base for psychiatric nursing. Almost single-handedly, she had set out to create a literature base for psychiatric nursing in the UK. There were many copies of Annie's book *Psychology for Nurses* at Tooting Bec Hospital and I can recall being told on several occasions that reading this book would be sufficient to enable any student to pass the two stages of the psychiatric nursing examination – the preliminary exam at the end of the first year and the final exam at the end of three years. In 1964, Una Budge organised a visit to the Maudsley School of Nursing to hear Annie talk on the history of the hospital. Annie struck me as business-like but friendly. Her reputation and the respect she evoked from her fellow-tutors appeared to mean less to her than her interest in the student nurses whose understanding of what the work of nursing consisted of, and why they had become nurses, she was keen to develop. She spoke fluently, without notes, and for the first time in my training, I heard someone talk about the anguish endured by those suffering from mental illness. She stressed that: 'We should never underestimate the power of human contact in ameliorating such suffering'. She was the first person I had heard speak of the unique role of psychiatric nursing, of the efficacy of human caring and of the significance of developing and sustaining helpful relationships with patients. She spoke of the Maudsley as a 'special place' where people felt understood and gained confidence that they could be helped. I remember how interested I was to learn that the hospital had evolved from a 13th century monastic foundation caring exclusively for people with mental illness. A minor observation I made on that visit was that the tutors at Tooting Bec wore white coats when they taught; Annie wore ordinary clothes. This spoke to me of her desire not to set herself apart, and perhaps of her need to be accepted as an `ordinary' person. It was obvious that Annie had a special affection for the Maudsley and those who worked there. Many years later, when she invited me to stay with her in Edinburgh, she talked again about the Maudsley and the impact made on her by those who worked there. She would bring me a cup of tea in bed every morning and would say, 'When you are up and awake, I have some interesting things to talk about that I have been thinking about during the night'.

As Ernest Hemingway once remarked, how our lives are to develop can be seen in their beginnings. Beginnings are critical. We can seek to deny them, accept them, or build on them, but we cannot ignore them. Our past is a part of our present and our future. It is my contention that while there is merit in trying to understand the `naked' text, knowledge of the biography of the author, in this case, Annie Altschul, enhances the text and leads to a deeper understanding of its meaning. We are the products of our biography as much as we are of our biology.

The Early Years

Annie Altschul was born in Vienna on 18th February 1919, the year the *Nurses Registration Act* was passed in England. Her father died suddenly when she was about two years old. She remembered her childhood as a carefree, happy time when her imagination was encouraged and her intellect stimulated. 'Life', she recalled later, 'was a gift that was time-limited, but held out endless possibilities for those who were able to take advantage of it'. Vienna between the wars was the epicentre of the cultured world, an intellectual vortex. The city could provide the best in terms of music, philosophy, medicine and psychiatry. The young Annie was wholeheartedly engaged with the city, where much of the life was driven by members of the Jewish community to which she belonged. The political climate was vibrant. Socialism was not merely venerated as an ideology, but was practised and manifest in the lives of ordinary people who enjoyed affordable housing, clean water, fresh air, public parks, museums, art galleries and other entertainments. Café life encouraged an ongoing exchange of ideas (as well as nurturing good business links!).

The social and intellectual environment of Annie Altschul's youth was one in which ideas came from and were owned by the people, and the essence of being human was located within and between people. The rich Vienna landscape, however, held mixed prospects of good and evil, for participating in the same café life as Annie and her friends were both the young Adolf Hitler and Albert Schweitzer. Very soon, the city which nurtured the fullness of people's humanity would resound to the thunder of marching armies, echo with foreign accents, and be swallowed up by those who placed no value on human life. At the end of the inter-war years, fear started to suppress the political and artistic energy and the free flow of ideas. Nazism and anti-Semitism grew daily stronger although few could envisage what was to happen.

Annie was naturally aware of the hill overlooking Vienna on which stood the Steinhof mental hospital. Over the main entrance, it was proclaimed that 'art and nature should come to the doors of the wards'. At that time, the hospital held little interest for her although, in her later life, she was to think much about its significance. The designer of the Steinhof was Vienna's foremost architect, Otto Wagner. Explaining the concept for his hospital,

Wagner commented: 'I wanted to bring into the hospital Viennese charm, joy and light and I wanted to avoid the clinical style that makes people feel locked-up'.

In 1938, when Annie was 19 years old and at university studying mathematics, Hitler forced the Austrian Chancellor, Kurt von Schuschnigg, to resign and installed Arthur von Seyss-Inquart, the leader of the Nazi Party in Austria, in his place. At the invitation of the Austrian Nazi Party, the German army marched into Austria and declared the union of Austria and Germany. The Munich Pact signed by Hitler, Mussolini, Chamberlain and Daladier of France gave the Sudetenland, the German speaking part of Czechoslovakia, to Germany. There followed almost immediately a day of violent rioting against the Jews known as the Kristallnacht (the night of broken glass). The attacks on the Jews were provoked largely by envy of their wealth and their control over the economic, business and cultural life of the country. In 1940, a convoy of German soldiers removed the 3000 patients from the Steinhof Hospital. Although the staff did what they could to resist, they could not prevent their patients being taken from the 'Golden Cage' to a killing centre near Linz. The hospital subsequently became the principal experimentation centre for the Nazis' eugenics policies in relation to sick children and the mentally ill from Austria and Germany (Glass, 2001).

A Refugee in England

In 1938, following in the footsteps of Sigmund Freud, Annie decided to leave Vienna and join her sister in England. What a departure that must have been - the urgency of the need to escape, the quandary about where she was going, and the uncertainty about what the future held! For Annie, as for others who have been displaced from their homes and native lands (e.g. Henry James, Albert Camus and Frank McCourt), living with displacement and uncertainty made her ultra-sensitive to what was happening around her.

When Annie arrived in England at the end of the 1930s, there were more than 50,000 Germans, Austrians and Czechoslovakians living in the UK. The Germans and the Austrians were classified as `enemy aliens'. They had to carry an 'Alien Registration Card' and report to the police regularly. They were forbidden to live or work in certain restricted areas. Anti-foreigner sentiment led to restrictions on employment. Annie recalled many years later that 'the extent of discrimination I experienced at that time was more painful than I ever thought possible, but at least I was alive and I had my mental faculties'.

Annie's first job in England was as a nanny to two pre-school children, but she soon gave this up to start work as a nurse at the Ealing Voluntary Hospital. In August 1940, there were an estimated 1000 unemployed nurses of enemy nationality living in England. Foreign qualifications were not accepted even though some professions, such as nursing, were desperate to recruit. Eventually, some hospitals started to employ these nurses and found them hard working, efficient and better educated than the indigenous nurses. At the General Lying-in Hospital in London and at the Royal Infirmary in Edinburgh, two Austrian refugees were taken on as midwives each year throughout the duration of the war. Further evidence that matrons were ignoring government directives is provided by a letter written in the summer of 1942 by the Chief Rabbi to the Matron of Claybury Hospital, an LCC institution, thanking her for granting leave to Jewish staff during holy days and requesting that she might do so again (John Stewart, personal communication).

As a result of the blitz, Annie moved to Surrey in 1940 and commenced her nurse training at Epsom County General Hospital. This she described as 'wartime training' - basic, no-nonsense, and frankly hostile to reflection or questioning on the part of students. It is hardly surprising, given that she had been forced to flee her own country and had received a somewhat hostile reception in this, that Annie felt drawn to the outsiders who came under her care, and especially to the gypsies who were regarded as inferior and excluded from the regular wards.

When she moved to Mill Hill to undertake psychiatric training, Annie felt as if it was a home-coming. Mill Hill Emergency Hospital had been set up by the Ministry of Health on the site of a former public school as a psychiatric centre for the treatment of military and civilian victims of shell-shock. It was staffed by members of the Maudsley Hospital and it was here that Maxwell Jones founded his therapeutic community. Many of the nurses were mature professional women who had chosen nursing as their contribution to the war effort. These women were accustomed to two-way communication, and not prepared simply to give orders to patients and receive them from doctors. Mill Hill provided an environment where people enjoyed being with people, talked to them, listened to them and were listened to in turn. Discussing patients, their problems, their progress and their futures with the most eminent people in the field, such as Emmanuel Millar, Maxwell Jones, Linford Rees, William Sargent, Elliot Slater and Aubrey Lewis was 'a sheer joy' to Annie. Here was the kind of vigorous intellectual climate which she had enjoyed in Vienna and she started to search for the theory and the literature that would enable her to help her patients most effectively. There was little, if any, to be found in the field of psychiatric nursing. On completing her psychiatric nurse training, Annie stayed on at the Maudsley as Staff Nurse and Sister until she was approached by Miss Olive Griffiths, the Assistant Matron, and invited to take responsibility for the School of Nursing. Soon after taking up her new post, Annie requested Reg Everest to join her and they formed a formidable partnership for almost a decade.

Post-War Travels

Annie went to the States from 1960 – 1961. She was not the first psychiatric nurse to travel overseas for professional purposes. During the 1950s, a group of psychiatric nurses from one of the Epsom hospitals had annually visited psychiatric hospitals in Holland and John Greene was awarded a travel scholarship to visit

Scandinavian hospitals in the early 1960s. Annie's visit was notable because of the length of her visit and the seniority of the visitor. She made substantial preparations beforehand, clarifying for herself the purpose of her journey and what she was hoping to achieve. She wanted to explore the nature of care and the experience of being cared for. Before she could do this, she felt she had to understand the culture in which care was provided:

'It is...impossible to understand the significance of a people's attitudes to work, to sickness, and to the [nursing] profession without love of its culture. Living in the USA for nearly a year, meeting people in their own homes, meeting their families, sharing with them leisure and work, enjoyment and anxieties, has helped me to understand a little more about the USA than I had before. I met many people in all walks of life, rich and poor, white and coloured, young and old...I met many people in no way connected with nursing and learnt a little about the way they view their health services and the nursing profession'. (Altschul, 1960:2001, p. 9)

And on another occasion, she wrote:

'I am well aware of the degree of security and the level of morale required to allow a complete stranger to participate in discussions of internal problems and I am deeply appreciative of the opportunity offered to me. Wherever I was able to meet patients and move freely among them, it was possible to gain some idea of staff-patient relationships'. (Altschul, 1960:2001, pp. 39-40)

While visiting state hospitals in California, Annie noticed that although resources of space, equipment and personnel appeared almost limitless, the philosophy, remit and nature of nursing were never discussed. Consequently, nursing care was poorly managed and poorly delivered. Nurses did not get to know their patients and patients could not develop a relationship with a particular nurse. Annie wondered why it was thought desirable or necessary to have toilets without doors and a total lack of privacy in the shower areas. The lives of old people seemed miserable. They had no special nurses to take an interest in them. The wards were large and institutionalised; all the counterpanes were alike; identical chairs stood in rows. The loneliness of patients was distressing. Affluence and democratic rhetoric did not necessarily translate into a caring environment even when carers were well-intentioned. Annie brought her own experiences of displacement to help her understand the impoverished social and spiritual lives of the patients.

Annie later spoke of how nothing had prepared her for what she experienced in some hospitals in America – an atmosphere redolent of dislike and disapproval of patients, and a complete absence of human sympathy. In such institutions, she found that staff meetings were simply an opportunity for nurturing ill feeling and exchanging ignorance. There was no sharing of insights into individual patients, and nurses had no interest in what they were doing. There was no attempt to deal with the problems of patients or staff through discussion. Annie reported how patients were permanently idle and bored, with no incentive to get out of bed in the morning or to attend to their personal appearance.

By contrast, attending the teaching sessions at the Boston University School of Nursing, and especially those of Dr. Apple, brought her the same 'sheer joy' that she had felt at Mill Hill. At the end of her time in Boston, she was full of admiration for the best in caring that was demonstrated there, while nonetheless feeling strong disappointment at the mediocrity of some of the students and their indifference to the learning opportunities available to them.

Annie's Report to the Commonwealth Fund on her study tour of the USA, Canada and Australia is a document that should act as a template for Reflective Practice. There one will find ample evidence of the range of her analytical skills, the acuteness of her perceptions, the vivacity of her curiosity and of her ability to immerse herself in every new experience. She was never afraid to criticise what she had seen and in her report on her time in America, disdained the kind of therapeutic relationships that are insincere and undertaken to gratify the self-esteem of one of the participants only.

Conclusion

Annie was a traveller throughout her life. She was a traveller who observed closely the people she met and the events happening around her. She was a traveller who was able to reflect with honesty and insight, evaluate, analyse and report on what she had learned in order to make her learning accessible to others. From her youth when she travelled from Vienna to London, and later in her life when she travelled to America, Canada, Australia and Singapore, she learnt that humanity is transmitted through relationships and that relationships can enhance humanness or diminish it. She was also a careful observer of her own experiences, and drew on them to help her understand the experiences of others. She understood the wisdom of the 'wounded healer' which we currently see driving the user movement. Annie was the first nurse in the UK to ask the fundamental questions about caring – What is the nature of caring? How it can be transmitted? What are the skills of the carer? She recognised the lack of any theoretical basis underpinning nursing and she dared to imagine what such a theory might look like, and to develop it. Her book, *Recent Advances in Psychiatric Nursing*, published by Churchill Livingstone in 1985 was one such contribution, in addition to countless journal articles.

Annie's background, combined with her intelligence, made her peculiarly sensitive to the world around her. For her, being displaced led to a life-long exploration of what kinds of human relationship promote comfort, solace and a sense of belonging. Experience of being the outsider drew Annie to other outsiders and she learned how to welcome them back into some kind of community. The greatness of her achievements is perhaps best summed up in the words of Laurens van der Post (1982) who noted that the ultimate in humanness is to be more than oneself; it is to be someone other. Although she was at times erratic, contemplative and effusive, she was always more than one expected her to be. Some may disagree, but I believe her greatest contribution to nursing and to those of us privileged to have known her was directed at the heart rather than the head.

References

Altschul, A. (1960:2001) 'Report on visits to state hospitals in California, etc. in June, July and August 1960' in Altschul, A. (2001) *A Festschrift for Annie Altschul.* Royal College of Nursing, Queen Margaret University College, and The University of Edinburgh.

Altschul, A. (1961:2001) 'Report on a tour of the United States of America, Canada and Australia to study psychiatric nursing: Report to the Commonwealth Fund' in Altschul, A. (2001) *A Festschrift for Annie Altschul.* Royal College of Nursing, Queen Margaret University College, and The University of Edinburgh.

Altschul, A. (2001) *A Festschrift for Annie Altschul.* Royal College of Nursing, Queen Margaret University College, and The University of Edinburgh.

Glass, N. (2001) 'The restoration of a historic hospital'. *The Lancet*, 357, 151-152

Van Der Post, L. (1982) *Yet Being Someone Other.* London: Penguin Books

Commentary 4

Developing practice: from the private to the public

David Glenister

David Glenister; Lecturer; School of Nursing, Social Work and Applied Health Studies; University of Hull

Introduction

The focus of this paper is the life of the 20th century's foremost British exponent of mental nursing, Emeritus Professor Annie Altschul CBE, FRCN, and addresses personal and public life. I will focus upon 'people who are nursed', specifically, Mrs. X., Miss Altschul, and myself. The primary sources used in this paper are the papers recently uncovered by Dr. Steve Tilley, Senior Lecturer, University of Edinburgh, which reported upon Miss Altschul's British Commonwealth for Nurses Scholarship Fund funded visit to the United States of America. I also draw upon my own interviews with Miss Altschul. While I was fumbling with tape recorder and cassettes Miss Altschul told me 'I am not a historian, but I have lived such a long time people come to speak to me about history' - one of those unrecorded casual reflections so frustrating to oral historians. There is, I wish to suggest, something to be learnt from Miss Altschul's personal reflections in public, that take us towards a fuller understanding of mental nursing, and perhaps even of being human in a complex world today.

The first part of this paper addresses the private

Mrs X

Miss Altschul did not accept Mrs. X's 'setting of the stage' for psychoanalytic psychotherapy, and refused the offer of a low armchair beside her bed. She offered instead, 'simply being together, enjoying companionship, liking each other' [Altschul 1960:2001a: 62]. For Mrs. X. this was 'second rate therapy' [Altschul 1960:

2001a:1].

Miss Altschul noted Mrs. X.'s 'inability to pursue emotional topics'. When Miss Altschul [1960:2001a:3] encouraged Mrs. X. to reflect upon herself, the result is 'verbal cliché, without emotion' [1960: 2001a:62]. 'It is obviously too difficult to look at herself. She blocks completely and says she cannot remember, or talks of her guilty feelings without evidence of feeling at all' [Altschul 1960:2001a: 63]. 'When anything approaches the topic of sex, she immediately stops talking altogether' [Altschul 1960:2001a:64]. 'She refers to her children's problems as it (sic) she were talking of case material' [Altschul 1960:2001a:63]. 'She blocks or changes subject, and with me found it easy to draw red herrings' [Altschul 1960:2001a:64]. Mrs. X. 'values material possessions for their own sake and professes interest in middle-class cultural values such as music, of which, however, she has no knowledge' [Altschul 1960:2001a:63].

Mrs. X is emotionally hollow, with only clichés, empty gestures and distractions to protect this inner emptiness. She does not know herself, or her feelings, especially her sexual feelings. She is unable to please herself, or others. Her social ambitions and materialism emphasise this hollowness. There is no secure sense of being, or being with others. Miss Altschul's exact prose reveals this emotional hollowness.

I wish nevertheless to suggest there is something of substance here that is not specified. This is alluded to in Miss Altschul's use of religious words, such as 'reverence'. Miss Altschul also refers to the 'new philosophy' of existentialism, but this is not referenced, or pursued. [In passing: Dr. R.D. Laing published *The Divided Self: An Existential Study in Sanity and Madness*, a few years earlier in 1959]. I wish to suggest the Jewish existentialist philosopher Martin Buber's work is useful here when attempting to articulate something so subtle yet so substantial.

Buber contrasted the 'eternal thou', with the limitations of things [Buber 1937]. Individuals could acknowledge the eternal thou in their relationships with others, and the eternal thou that transcended all individuals. This would also involve individuals ceasing to use each other as things. This acknowledgement, or turning, could transform individuals and institutions. The eternal thou could transform the hollow world of things to the hallowed world of thou in relation to thou. Miss Altschul acknowledged the hollowness of Mrs. X, but there was no transformation. Despite this, I wish to suggest her combination of existentialism and religious language promises something more.

To grasp something so substantial yet so subtle, I wish to move beyond the texts, and the hints within them, to my own experience of Miss Altschul.

There was a time, almost two years ago now, when I experienced unspeakable terror, and was beyond everyday reality. Miss Altschul invited me to stay for a weekend, after I had written to her at the suggestion of a friend. She wrote back indicating that she knew of my aloneness, and suggested I was disturbed and deluded. Afterwards, I wrote of my understanding of the relationship between mental health and mental illness.

Mental illness and mental health are not mutually exclusive, since one can be deeply depressed, even beyond standard reality, and yet more true to oneself, more true to others, than one has even had the courage to be before. Thus, mental illness, in the form of psychosis, and mental health, in the sense of a terrifying and exotic authenticity can exist together, in the same person, in the same time, in the same place [Glenister 1999].

The issue here for me was that of being authentic in the world, and the awful realization of inauthenticity. This realization was terrifying.

To be truly sick is to discover health, and this necessarily involves a savage tearing of the veil of illusions, the petty illusions and lies of one's life story, and the bigger illusions and lies of the world in which most of us live, most of the time. This rape of innocence is a disgusting and desperate act, yet it is necessary if we are to move beyond both private and public non-reality. Whether an act courted, or threatened and then endured is somewhat irrelevant. To enjoy the wineglass of blood red wine of life to the full, one must taste, and even learn to enjoy, the last mouthful of foul and fetid dregs [Glenister 1999].

To be nursed, I discovered, was to discover the authentic within the inauthentic.

I found being nursed humiliating and hurtful, not because of her, but because she left me alone with my own torment. No cloying words of comfort, but the simple acknowledgement of the way things were. A simple refusal of lies and illusions. Few words were said, for we mostly spoke and listened telepathically, sometimes when I was awake, and sometimes when I was asleep. She was like a mirror, in which my deformities were starkly exposed. She simply was. Profoundly reconciled to herself and the world, yet aware of the possibility of change [Glenister 1999].

I have taken the rather unusual step of the disclosure of the personal in public because it may reveal something of Miss Altschul's mental nursing practice. Authentic being, resolute ontology, was, and indeed still is, it appears to me, central to Miss Altschul's mental nursing practice. This is a severe challenge to the ontological insecurity to be found in mental illness, as indicated in Dr. Laing's [1959] early work. This conflict between one's own ontological insecurity and someone else's relative ontological security is greatly disturbing. However, there is something ultimately satisfying in discovering something trustworthy within, of finding something hallowed rather than hollow.

The second part of the paper addresses making private knowledge public

The content of Miss Altschul's [1985] contribution to *The*

Wounded Healer is mostly unremarkable in its lack of detail of the experience of mental illness, and mental nursing and its style. There is a intimation of 'very real and overwhelming personal problems' [Altschul 1985:168], but there is a tacit agreement that the past will not be discussed [Altschul 1985:170], and good nursing is described as little more than tactful observation to ensure safety, the serving of tea, accompanied walks, and the inevitable game of Scrabble [Altschul 1985:170]. At best, nurses were 'respectful', and 'never condescending' [Altschul 1985:170]. There is no suggestion of constructive conversations, other than 'small talk' [Altschul 1985: 170], but as indicated above sometimes physical and psychological presence can be affirming, or few words, or even no words. This text indicates again the difficulty of writing about nursing, its substance not being articulated even by the seasoned observer, such as Miss Altschul.

The existence of the chapter is nevertheless remarkable, for it is a public discussion of private events; more particularly, in its discussion of psychiatric patienthood by someone who was at the time an esteemed professional. Altschul revealed herself not just as someone who studied and taught mental illness, but as someone who for a time was mentally ill. This was a subversion of the public proper.

A comparison is helpful here to reveal the situation. Another nurse tutor, Ms. Mary Barnes, who died this year, was the most famous resident of Kingsley Hall, where she undertook a journey to the depths of madness and back. Ms. Mary Barnes and Dr. Jo Burke, influenced by Dr. R. D. Laing, sought to understand recovery from psychosis and schizophrenia. This famously involved not only a breakdown of standard reality, but a breakthrough to a new ontologically sounder reality. Later, Ms. Mary Barnes herself established a refuge for those in emotional turmoil. She was, like Miss Altschul, a missionary into madness. It is of note that both Miss Annie Altschul and Ms. Mary Barnes were women who sought to turned their private pain into public politics. This personification contrasts with that traditionally male prerogative of pontificating.

Dr. R. D. Laing, for example, a most eloquent speaker, never moved beyond the quagmire of his own despair [Huxley 2001].

The third part of the paper addresses psychiatric politics

English social psychiatry: Altschul wrote of California 'our concept of Social Psychiatry has great appeal', and specifically mentioned a forthcoming visit by Maxwell Jones [Altschul 1961/2001:21]. This is elaborated when topics of discussion are noted in the California visit

Among topics most frequently raised, apart from questions about England, were problems related to Ward Management, Therapeutic Community and Patient Government [Altschul 1960b/2001: 40]

Miss Altschul's use of the possessive case, 'our concept of Social Psychiatry' tellingly denotes both national and therapeutic affinities.

The development of democratic psychiatric services, and the critique of authoritarianism is evident in the California report [Altschul 1960:9], and owes much to the work of Dr. Eric Fromm, and the largely Jewish refugees of the Frankfurt School in exile. Dr. Hildegard Peplau was supervised by Dr. Fromm [Barker 1998], and his influence upon her work is readily evident, in its focus upon patients developing skills in participating in wards, hospitals and society at large.

In his American history of psychiatry, Shorter [1997] referred to social psychiatry as the English contribution to global psychiatry. This is an understandable mistake. Dr. Joshua Bierer, Dr. Maxwell Jones, Dr. J.R. Rees and Dr. T.P. Rees, the most prominent proponents, were resident in England, but not English. Dr. J.R. Rees and Dr. T.P. Rees were Welsh, and Maxwell Jones was a South African, of Welsh descent, who was resident in Scotland at the outbreak of war. Dr. Joshua Bierer, like Miss Altschul, was a Jewish refugee. His contribution to English social psychiatry was the establishment of Marlborough Day Hospital, democratic Social

Clubs [later to evolve into Clubhouses], and self-help networks. Nevertheless, his work has been largely ignored in the history of social psychiatry. Until Shorter [1997] his place within the history of psychiatry is almost entirely marginal. His eccentricity, grandiosity and thick Germanic accent may not have helped in this matter [Clarke 1998], but nor can his status as a Jewish refugee be discounted as irrelevant.

Mental nurses were central to social psychiatry, because they were integral to the 'therapeutic environment', but not to consulting room psychotherapeutic psychiatry. Their role was not 'thought out' in the latter, but had been in the former [Altschul 1961:2001: 21]. There can be little doubt that Miss Altschul sought to 'think out' the role of the nurse in social psychiatry. As such, she was one of its chief practitioners and propagandists, and this becomes more remarkable when the general absence of women in the history of psychiatry is considered. Despite this, Altschul does not yet have a place in the history of social psychiatry. This may simply be a matter of not being a psychiatrist, but then being a Jewish woman may be relevant too.

A public and political life After the Second World War Altschul was an active member of the Socialist Medical Association, and relished the company of other socialists. Unlike Dr. Peplau, who briefly under the influence of Eric Fromm criticised authoritarian practices and advocated democratic practice but thereafter sought the narrower aims of ensuring nurses were not second class citizens [Lego 1999], Miss Altschul remained faithful to her early political vision.

In British 20th century mental nursing, it is not easy to find a peer of anything like Miss Altschul's standing. There is nevertheless one individual who shared her socialist commitments, political aptitude, and willingness to enter the public sphere in pursuit of political aims, namely, Mr. George Gibson. English eugenic legislation was presented in 1931 by Major Church, but unlike the German legislation two years later relied upon voluntary rather than involuntary sterilization, and did not address penal cases [Blacker 1933-4]. Mr. Gibson, as General Secretary of National Asylum Workers Union [NAWU], and Dr. Hyacinth Morgan, a NAWU-sponsored MP, played significant roles in defeating this legislation [Carpenter 1988]. Dr. Blacker [1952-3:17], the General Secretary of the Eugenics Society, later undertook a study of German National Socialist eugenics and vivisection. He concluded that 'on a scale of moral turpitude, the euthanasia of the insane ranks lower than the vivisection of human beings' and that 'the principle of the inviolability of human life goes by the board in war time...when human life is held cheap' but acts of 'vivisection of human beings' were 'atrocities'. The defeat of the British 1931 eugenic legislation was perhaps a defining moment in the history of mental nursing, when an alliance of the trade union movement and the labour movement sought to defend the working class, and individuals with disabilities within it.

Before the *Nurses Act 1943*, Mr. Gibson thwarted the attempt to introduce the second-level mental nurse, while Mrs. Bedford-Fenwick failed in the same endeavour with regard to the second level general nurse. In 1945 Mr. Gibson sought to establish undergraduate and post-graduate nurse education, including doctoral nurse education, and to link grading with education. Mr. Gibson rose to become the General Secretary of the Trades Union Congress, arguably the most prestigious and powerful post within the male working class public sphere. These two individuals shared a commitment to socialism and an opposition to eugenics. One working class male, one middle class female; one sought the occupational advancement of mental nursing through trade unionism and the other through academia. The routes taken by these two individuals into the public sphere were structured within gendered and classed opportunities.

The public and the private: Several boundaries between the public and the private have been examined in the paper. First, the fluid boundary between spiritual and temporal time, the former involving the covenantal authentic acknowledgement of thou, sometimes even transcendence of time itself, and the acknowledgement of things in contractual clock time. This fluid boundary has been recently explored by Tilley and Pollock [1999]. Second, disruptions to the boundary of private pain and public politics. Two women have been described who disrupted the boundary between private and public through their assumption of patienthood, one temporarily and one almost permanently. The notion of redemptive sacrifice cannot be ignored here. Thirdly, the more stable geographical boundaries between social class-based and gendered spheres. The occupational opportunities for advancement of a middle class woman were addressed. The absence of women in the almost entirely male history of psychiatry was noted. The specific difficulties faced by Jewish refugees in medicine and nursing were also noted briefly. In short, the boundaries between private and public can be demarcated by time, feeling and thought and geography, and these boundaries cannot be separated from considerations of class, gender, and religion. Summers [2000:18] usefully argues that when women [such as Miss Altschul] entered public life they brought with them into the public sphere formerly private traditions, such as the covenant rather than the contract, and the spiritual rather than the secular. 'Lineages' [Summers [2000:18] transmitted these traditions. I do not mean to appear discourteous when I suggest Miss Altschul's work may at present be most sympathetically received by migrants, emigrés, and others who have crossed boundaries.

The fourth part of the paper addresses epistemology

Living the past in the present the historian seeks to discover the past in its remnants. Usually these remnants of the past are material, e.g. documents, tape recordings and badges. However, these remnants are also mentalities. These mentalities have a continued existence, more subtle yet stronger than material remnants. Historians in a sense are the living past, just as others of today are, but the difference is that historians seek to know the past they live.

Before presenting themselves as master craftsmen of stories made out of the past, historians must stand as heirs to the past. This idea of inheritance presupposes that the past in some sense lives in the present and therefore affects it. It is this passive dimension of historical inheritance that is best expressed by the idea of historical debt. Before even forming the idea of re-presenting the past, we are in debt to the men and women of the past who contributed to making us what we are. Before we can represent the past we must live as beings affected by the past [Ricoeur 1981:23:italics in original].

Thus Ricoeur indicates the primacy of ontology, of temporal being in this world, and from this follows an epistemology which seeks to acknowledge the lives of the living past. In this paper, I have attempted to work reflexively, drawing upon my own struggle towards humanity in the presence of a humane other, and at the same time to address social and political realities.

Conclusion

As a nurse historian, I am conscious of Ricoeur's emphasis upon the idea of historical debt, and I have attempted to make a small payment against this debt by attempting to articulate the relationship between the private and the public. The crossing of boundaries, between the private and the public, has formed a theme in this paper about the life of Emeritus Professor Miss Altschul CBE, FRCN. These boundaries have been between the sacred and secular, the public and the personal, and classed and gendered social spheres. These boundaries have formed the background to Miss Altschul's daily search for the authentic spiritually hallowed within the inauthentic emotionally hollow. That this is the life of a Jewish socialist middle class woman refugee cannot be ignored, and indeed this personal experience may have informed many public actions. Reverence for words and books, and the importance of ensuring that reverence is appropriately placed, is explicitly indicated in Miss Altschul's report upon her visit to the United States of America, and perhaps without her lifelong search for reverant words of substance we would not be meeting here today.

References

Altschul, A. (1960/2001a) 'Report on the one-to-one relationship with Mrs. X, Boston', Pages 61-64 IN Altschul, A. (2001) *A Festschrift for Annie Altschul,* Department of Nursing Studies, The University of Edinburgh, and UK Centre for the History of Nursing.

Altschul, A. (1960b/2001) Report on visits to state hospitals in California etc. in June, July and August 1960. Pages 37-49 IN Altschul, A. (2001) *A Festschrift for Annie Altschul,* Department of Nursing Studies, The University of Edinburgh, and UK Centre for the History of Nursing.

Altschul, A. (1961:/2001) Report on a tour of the United States of America, Canada and Australia to study psychiatric nursing. May 1960-April 1961. Report to the Commonwealth Fund. Pages 2-36 IN Altschul, A. (2001) *A Festschrift for Annie Altschul,* Department of Nursing Studies, The University of Edinburgh, and UK Centre for the History of Nursing.

Altschul, A. (1985) 'There won't be a next time', Pages 167-175 IN Rippere, V. & Williams, R. (eds.) (1985) *Wounded healers: mental health workers' experiences of depression,* John Wiley, Chichester.

Blacker, C.P. (1952-3) 'Eugenic' experiments conducted by the Nazis upon human subjects, *Eugenics Review* 22 9-19.

Buber, M. (1937) *I and Thou* Trans. Smith, R. G. Edinburgh: T and T Clark

Burleigh, M. (1994) *Death and Deliverance: 'Euthanasia' in Germany 1900-1945,* Cambridge: Cambridge University Press

Carpenter, M. [1988] *Working for Health: the history of the Confederation Of Health Service Employees,* London: Laurence and Wishart

Clarke, L. (1997) 'Joshua Bierer: Striving for Power', *History of*

Psychiatry, viii, 319-332.

Glenister, D. (1999) 'Discovering health in sickness', Hull: Unpublished Paper

Huxley, F. (2001) 'Shamanism, Healing and R.D. Laing': The Second R. D. Laing Conference Royal College of Psychiatrists: Philosopy Special Interest Group Saturday 21 October 2000 London: School of Oriental and African Studies

Laing, R. D. (1959) *The Divided Self: An Existential Study in Sanity and Madness*, London: Tavistock Books

Lego, S. (1996) 'Psychoanalysis and Psychiatric Nursing in America. An historical and current perspective', Association of Psychoanalytic Psychotherapy Conference, "The Culture of Nursing:Psychoanalytic Perspectives". October 12, 1996, Tavistock Clinic, London.

Ricour, P. (1981) *Hermeneutics and the Human Sciences*, [Trans. J.B. Thompson] Cambridge: Cambridge University Press

Shorter, E. (1997) *A History of Psychiatry: From the Era of the Asylum to the Age of Prozac*, New York: John Wiley and Sons

Summers, A. (2000) *Female Lives, Moral States: Women, Religion and Public Life 1800-1930*, Newbury: Threshold Press

Tilley, S. and Pollock, L. (1999) The two cultures of the Community Psychiatric Nurse: 'twixt contract and covenant in work with 'people with enduring mental disorders', Paper presented at the 22nd International Council of Nurses Congress, London, 29-6-99.

Commentary 5

Annie Altschul and the Austro-Hungarian Matrix – the individual and the group

Phil Barker

Phil Barker PhD RN FRCN; Visiting Professor, Trinity College Dublin. Email: Phil_Barker@ukf.net

A day when Fuji
Is obscured by misty rain!
That's interesting.
(Basho)

[Note: Annie Altschul is no more or less than a remarkable story. When asked to present at the festschrift I chose not to write a formal paper, as requested, but instead to bring a few thoughts about Annie that I could use as the basis for developing another story about her and the story of her life and work. This is the story that emerged.]

I did not bring a formally prepared paper with me to this festschrift. As I began to think, a moment ago, about what I had brought with me, it occurred to me that it was something akin to a 'dark glass'. Some renaissance artists reputedly developed a device to reflect an image through a sheet of glass painted black. The device was meant to enable the artist to see more clearly, paradoxically, through the darkness. They assumed that the brilliance of natural light made it difficult to see what was, literally, in their line of vision. As I listened to the other speakers, I began to think that I had brought a kind of dark glass to serve as a reflection of Annie's texts. I do not intend to refer to her work directly but, instead, bring some of my personal, heartfelt reflections on her writing, and try to set these in context, framed by observations others have made about her and her work.

The story, which is emerging here, in my view, concerns an understanding of the Self: the person who becomes the patient, or the client, or the user, or consumer, or whatever we are calling them in this strange world of mental health, other than simply persons. When I re-read Annie's papers, I was reminded of Alan Watts, the heretical English theologian, who went to the USA and, at the same time as Annie visited, began to establish himself as the guru of my generation. Watts' great contribution was to help us appreciate the possible parallels between ancient Oriental thought and Western philosophy. Watts' contribution to the study of comparative philosophy, spirituality and theology, established him as an icon of the Me Generation. When reading Annie's thoughts about what she encountered on that first trip to the US, I was reminded of a book that Watts (1964) wrote around this time called *Beyond Theology*. In his opening, Watts asked, "who is the I who is me?" For Watts, the answer was like a Chinese box. The inherent riddle of the Self – who is the I who is me? - concerns the strangest kind of personal epistemology, which Watts illustrated in his answer:

'Is it the I who knows (who I am), or is the I who knows that I know, or is it the I who knows that I know that I know?'

Within the metaphor of the Chinese box, this question continues, *ad infinitum*. Watts was trying to convey, albeit obliquely, his appreciation that the Self was a Western construction, a point to which I shall return later. However, it seems clear that Annie's concern about the nature of what was going on, within the interpersonal exchanges that she was observing, and which were framed by Hildegard Peplau's interpersonal relations theory (Peplau, 1952), embraced at least something of the same kind of wonder about the nature of the thing Peplau referred to as the Self.

I have referred in the title of my paper to the Austro-Hungarian matrix. Today, people often ask – where is the 21st century Mozart? – acknowledging that the Central European world, (which many located around and about the Austro-Hungarian Empire), was the seed bed for many great minds, great art, and many great understandings about what it meant to be human. Many of those products and ideas have become enmeshed with our appreciation of what we call, 'Western culture'. Today, however, in a post-modern context, much of this tradition is dismissed as a 'Eurocentric' view of the world.

I know three people, each of whom when I asked them to tell me where their roots lay, located themselves within 50 to 100 miles of one another in that old Austro-Hungarian Empire. One is the great Antichrist of psychiatry – Tom Szasz. Some years ago, we were having a drink in the bar at a conference, and he was telling me a story about how he had left Budapest as a young man of 19, to go to the USA, possessing not a single word of English. He had only recently returned there with his family, having vowed never to go back as long as it was under communist rule. As he talked eloquently and vibrantly about his return to his homeland, I asked him "so Tom, would you describe yourself as an Hungarian?" He laughed and in his typically engaging manner said:

'Ah, a very good question, Phil. Do I think of myself as an Hungarian? No. Now if you had asked me do I think of myself as an American, I also would have said no! I am not an American. I am not an Hungarian. I am me!'

In that moment I understood Tom Szasz's fascination over the past 50 years, indeed some would say, obsession, with personal responsibility and liberty.

Hildegard Peplau was, in more than one sense of the word, a neighbour of Tom Szasz. Although born in the USA her family stemmed from the same central European territory. Once, when I asked her to try to sum up her theory of interpersonal relations, in the context of the generation and resolution of human problems, Hilda drew long and hard on her cigarette and said "people make themselves up as they talk". I have never been able to find that statement in her vast writings, but that seemed to represent an eloquent distillation of everything that she had been trying to say, down the years, about the importance of discourse: how humans come to know who they are. 'Who is the I who is me?'

The third person whom I know, whose roots lie in that Austro-Hungarian matrix is of course Shirley Smoyak. I have tried on numerous occasions to ask her 'Who is Shirley Smoyak?' but have never got a reasonable answer. Perhaps, of course, that was an answer. I was hoping that I might be able to ask her again here today, in open court if you like, but regrettably she cannot be with us, other than in spirit.

What is important about this Austro-Hungarian matrix has been very usefully prepared for me by Peter Nolan's wonderful evocation of the political and social factors that led to Annie's departure from her homeland and arrival here in the UK. What appears to me to be fundamental to Annie's wrestling with understanding - which characterised some of her commentaries about her American trip – involves ideas about the nature of the world that clearly stem from the intellectual melting pot of her homeland. I shall return to this later when I talk about the crucible of experience, for Annie Altschul's work is fundamentally about experience. David Glenister has offered a fine introduction to what I have to say about this, with his references to Mary Barnes, Kingsley Hall and Ronnie Laing. These are signposts, if you like, for other people – like Annie – who were trying to get close to the crucible of experience, without getting too badly burned in the process.

Not long after Annie's entry into nursing, she began to tussle with the question, 'what is it that one needs to do, to support people who are in some kind of state of madness'. I was very cheered a few years back that Annie acknowledged the virtue and value of the term madness, as more meaningful and descriptive of what she, herself, had experienced (Altschul, 1999). Certainly she thought this term was preferable to the political correctness that had been imported to try to soften the blow of what is called, socially, mental illness. In the early days of the war, she had begun to explore ways of coming to some kind of understanding of what that madness might be about. In the context of our discussion here today, it was no accident that she was fumbling with those understandings under blitz conditions. She came to find herself in these chaotic conditions, having escaped the chaos that reigned in her homeland. I think also that it was no accident that Annie found comfort, and a place in the world, in the emergent therapeutic communities of places like Mill Hill. Here there was a sense of doing things together. I intend no disrespect to the Peplauvian paradigm that emerged from interpersonal relations theory, but the emphasis on the golden hour of therapy – this almost paranoid focus on the interaction between one person defined as therapeutic agency and the other defined as patient – differed greatly from the stories that Annie has shared with me about her experience of being with, and living with, people who were patients in those blitz-torn hospitals in London.

She once told me about how she used to enter the hospital through a door in a wall, which was one of the few walls left standing in that part of the hospital. Ironically, it had no roof. So, in a sense, the community that lived within it was a kind of 'institution without walls' (or at least without a roof). It was there that she also began to appreciate the virtue and value of chance meetings and chance associations. Perhaps this reflects the great distinction between what emerged from Altschul's work, which 'naturally' favoured the broad social context, and the Peplauvian paradigm, with its emphasis on the 'intimacy' of the one-to-one relationship. Perhaps it was this appreciation of the value of chance happenings which disturbed Shirley Smoyak when she was frustrated by Annie's desire to go on a journey that had no goals. Shirley's is, of course, a curiously American frustration, given the heavily goal-directed nature of their society.

I recall also once, Annie referring to her memory of working with a woman who was, in her words, 'the craziest woman I had met, then or since'. Annie was sitting with this woman, day in and day out, trying to make sense of what she was saying – which was referred to in medical textbooks as 'word salad'. She had a flash of understanding one day when she realised that after spending time with this woman by day, she went home at night and tried to read (and understand) James Joyce. She realised that both Joyce and this woman, were talking in the same voice, although telling very different stories. This is another example of the chance insight that stems from the chance encounter.

Someone who has not been mentioned, and who was very important to her, was Annie's brother, who went to a kibbutz, largely as a function of his socialist persuasion. This chance happening also represents an important connection, as Annie's enthusiasm for ideas like the therapeutic community may, in a sense, also be 'in the blood'. More importantly, this is also part of the importance of the existential tradition, which was alluded to, but not picked up strongly in her writings on the trip.

Existentialism is, arguably, best represented by the writings and thought of Nietzsche, who was a fervent atheist; Buber, who was a powerful, if unconventional theologian; and Sartre who, although not a fully paid-up member, had strong communist sympathies. Existentialism, therefore, had numerous influences, most of which were disparate and disjointed. It is no surprise that the kind of existentialism to which Annie Altschul was attracted, was chaotic and uncertain. That uncertainty was perhaps the feature that was most attractive to her. It is also notable that Ronnie Laing was attracted to existentialism for many of the same reasons, in particular the Nietzschean, Buberian and Sartrian elements. Daniel Burston (2000), in his recent biography of Laing, acknowledged the existential basis of all of Laing's work, noting that

'Existentialism stresses that, despite disparate social and historical contexts, differences in age, gender, ability etc, all people, by virtue of their mortality, partake of the same basic structure of existence (Burston calls this 'throwness'– where life's contingencies result in the need to infuse or confer value and to impart meaning to life, through actions and decisions – thus taking responsibility for our personal destiny.'

I think that Annie Altschul would have been very comfortable in Kingsley Hall. What many people find discomforting about Kingsley Hall are just the things that would have made it very comfortable for her - especially the highly uncertain nature of the social milieu. Again, if she had been here, I would have loved to ask her, but I suspect that Shirley Smoyak would have been massively uncomfortable at Kingsley Hall – lacking as it did the structure, the goal-directedness, and the neurotic concern with doing something to some particular purpose. Altschul seemed to be more concerned with finding out, than in pursuing some predetermined objective.

There have already been references to the *Wounded Healer* (Rippere and Williams, 1985). Again, in the context of "who is the I who is me?", autonomy is very much part of the Altschul journey. One of the very interesting features of the *Wounded Healer* text was that Annie was one of only two people to put their name to their chapters. As far as Annie was concerned there was no embarrassment in admitting to having been in some state that might be called madness. This offers a poignant echo for the reference to Harry Stack Sullivan in Shirley Smoyak's paper. It is worth pointing out the little-known fact that Sullivan was largely marginalized by the American psychiatric community on the basis that he was probably as mad as his patients (Evans, 1996). I was told by a student of Sullivan that Sullivan was the first analyst to take his chair from behind the patient (analysand) and to draw it up alongside the patient. From that simple gesture, I believe, has flowed a whole series of developments that take us to our interests today in collaboration, empowerment and partnership in care. Despite the attempts to sideline Sullivan, his consideration of the power relationship appears to have long outlived him.

Annie Altschul was certainly someone who was interested in sitting alongside the patient (rather than opposite the patient as in the Peplauvian tradition) to begin to negotiate a relationship that was potentially confrontational, but certainly goal-directed in nature. In that sense Altschul was far more interested in journeying with the patient, than in taking them anywhere, if you like, by the hand.

I was particularly taken by Annie's reference in her text to her awareness that, were she to become a nurse in America she would prefer to be a nursing aide, rather than a registered nurse. That was entirely typical of my experience of this woman who remains an enigma. Annie Altschul is the laughing buddha of psychiatric nursing – she is inscrutable. If someone were to ask me what she stands for, I would find it very difficult to be concise, which perhaps explains why I have wandered around the houses here today. There is, however, an echo in what I have had to say.

Let us return to my opening remarks about how the Self comes to be, and how the self becomes disturbed and damaged. Alan Watts' typically Zen observation on the mind was that it was like ripples on a lake. The ripples are part of the thing called the lake but also a function of something far beyond, indeed removed from, the lake. The mind of Annie Altschul is not encased within her body, neither is it encased within her cultural heritage. The mind of Annie Altschul is in this room today and is also in the hearts and minds of people I have met, as far away as Australia and New Zealand, who have been influenced by her work and the thinking within it.

References

Altschul, A. (1999) 'Foreword' in P. Barker, P. Campbell and B. Davidson (eds.) *From the Ashes of Experience: Reflections on madness, recovery and growth*, London: Whurr.

Burston, D. (2000) *The crucible of experience: RD Laing and the crisis of psychotherapy*, Cambridge Mass: Harvard University Press.

Evans, F. B. (1996) *Harry Stack Sullivan: Interpersonal theory and psychotherapy*, London: Routledge.

Peplau, H. E. (1952) *Interpersonal relations in nursing*, New York: Putnam.

Watts, A. (1964) *Beyond Theology: The art of godmanship*, New York: Pantheon.

Commentary 6

'Gifts of argument, relationship, and tradition: boons of re-reading Altschul'

Stephen Tilley

Stephen Tilley PhD BA RMN; Senior Lecturer Nursing Studies; School of Health in Social Science; University of Edinburgh 31 Buccleuch Place, Edinburgh EH8 9JT, email: s.tilley@ed.ac.uk

Introduction

This is my reading of Annie Altschul's 1960-61 texts relating to her visit to the United States.

I want to focus this reading on Annie's practices of reading and re-reading, as I find them represented in these texts. My reading of Annie's texts focuses on:

- the value of reading and re-reading, *for Annie*

- the value of reading and re-reading parts of *Annie's work* (these texts the example) in the context of her other work

- more generally the value of (and the tradition of) *reading and re-reading texts in psychiatric nursing*

The value of reading and re-reading for Annie

Reading helped Annie solve a practical problem: how to teach psychiatric nursing to a new variety of students. Reading Greenblatt *et al* (1955), she had a 'bible', an authoritative text, which she drew on in her work as teacher. That text indicated that there were prospects of answering her questions about teaching if she went to the source, Boston, and the sources, including – especially - June Mellow. Mellow is presented as an exemplar of psychiatric nursing practice and teaching in Greenblatt *et al.* Reading Greenblatt *et al*'s text, Annie was promised a wider scope for learning and developing teaching and practice.

Reading Greenblatt *et al* perhaps also suggested what to do to solve the problem: *go out, to find out.* Leave the familiar, and unquestioned practice, and go to another place where practice had been questioned and changed. Greenblatt *et al* offered, or promised, that.

Greenblatt *et al*, we surmise, provided some sense of a *tradition* (*viz.* the 'bible' metaphor) and an *interpretive schema* for understanding practice, for making sense of what psychiatric nursing might be.

I here draw on MacIntyre's notions of 'tradition', and 'interpretive schema'.

'For the story of my life is always embedded in the story of those communities from which I derive my identity...What I am...is in key part what I inherit, a specific past that is present to some degree in my present. I find myself part of a history and that is generally to say, whether I like it our not, whether I recognize it or not, one of the bearers of a tradition.' (MacIntyre, *After Virtue*, p 221)

'...when a tradition is in good order it is always partially constituted by an argument about the goods the pursuit of which gives to that tradition its particular point and purpose.' (p. 222)

'A living tradition then is an historically extended, socially embodied argument, and an argument precisely in part about the goods which constitute that tradition.' (p. 222)

Again, MacIntyre writes:

'[What] constitutes a tradition is a conflict of interpretations of that tradition, a conflict which itself has a history susceptible of rival interpretations. If I am a Jew, I have to recognise that the tradition of Judaism is partly constituted by a continuous argument over what it means to be a Jew.' (p 249) [1]

For MacIntyre a tradition provides some means and methods for resolving questions and arguments about truth claims – e.g. about the appropriate role of the nurse and the value of one-to-one relationships between patients and nurses.

Taking MacIntyre's stance, we can say that reading, for Altschul, provided a sense of the goods of psychiatric nursing practice and education. Greenblatt *et al* were read as indicating that these goods had been realised in Boston, in the work of June Mellow. That text, and that reading, provided a sense of relationship to a tradition.

The narrative in Greenblatt *et al*, about practice in Boston, provided the stimulus for Annie to undertake a real trip with the aim of taking her practice *further*. That trip generated the narrative in Annie's 1960-61 text.

The value of reading and re-reading Annie's work

The narrative of travel and the quest: The texts document her travels. I read them as exemplars of great travel writing and more importantly, participant observation. The participant observer involves herself in the setting she comes to, but keeps self sufficiently disengaged, or uninvolved, to observe. It is the role of the not-wholly-committed.

Through her texts, Annie takes us into a reality, a culture, a

---

[1] I am a nurse, I have to recognise that the tradition of nursing is partly constituted by a continuous argument over what it means to be a nurse. The BU papers can then be seen as argument over what it is to be a nurse: focusing on argument (don't accept one view of what it is – anti-monolithic; use critique of US nurses not arguing). Relationship (what kind? with whom?, for whom?), tradition (Annie going at the particular point where 'school' was becoming 'discipline' was becoming 'institution' [see Tilley and Ryan, 2004]?)

people.

She also takes us readers on a *quest*. I see the broad narrative of these texts as a version of the quest story. Her quest, like all, is to answer questions. But through the quest the real questions are found. And the answers are implicit in those found questions.

Aspects of the quest: Here I draw on Andrea Hulme's (1991) account of aspects of the quest. 'The main protagonist, quester or hero undertakes a journey which is realised on both an external, physical level and in terms of inner reflectiveness.' We can see the first (external and physical) part in Annie's account of her 'external' travels to and in the US and the activities she undertook (including the one-to-one relationship formed with Mrs. X). The second journey (cf. Bruner's 'internal landscape') is discerned in the *reflexivity* of Annie's account of the travel and its meanings. 'A quest,' says MacIntyre, 'is always an education both as to the character of that which is sought and in self-knowledge.' [2]

According to Hulme, the quest has three stages:

1) starting out

2) the ordeals leading to the acquisition of the reward

3) return [3]

---

[2] 'The unity of a human life is the unity of a narrative quest...A quest for what? Two key features of the medieval conception of a quest need to be recalled. The first is that without some at least partly determinate conception of the final *telos* there could not be any beginning to a quest. Some conception of the good for man is required...Secondly it is clear...in the course of the quest and only through encountering and coping with the various particular harms, dangers, temptations and distractions which provide any quest with its episodes and incidents that the goal of the quest is finally to be understood. A quest is always an education both as to the character of that which is sought and in self-knowledge.' (MacIntyre, *After Virtue)*

[3] 'The first of the quest stages begins with an initial separation of the main quester

Questions serve to guide the hero 'along an unknown path which will reveal itself only as they progress:[4]

'What is the meaning of this?

What can it lead me to?

What can it teach me?

What is it to serve?' (Hulme, 1991)

The narrative of the U.S. visit: I read Annie's texts as documents of a quest in which original aims are lost sight of; and as documents of a process of mixing up of *what is* and *what seems*. They are thus documents of an epistemological crisis.

From one perspective, they are exemplary documents of methodical inquiry. Findings produced through participant observation contradict what Annie thought to be the case. She undertakes a series of smaller and larger 'experiments' to test her understanding and perception against reality.

Annie's main way of knowing is through involvement as participant observer – involve yourself but keep part of yourself out. She

---

from his/her accustomed reality...The quest is initiated by some kind of radical or painful split in their world which heralds a change in their once stable relationship with their surroundings.' For Annie, the change was associated with the need to teach a different group of nurses in a different way. This was one change in stable relationships with her surroundings. Another was the change from her setting of practice, on going to the US. Another was the change from the one-removed picture of a different kind of practice – the image of psychiatric and psychiatric nursing practice she had from Greenblatt *et al* – to moving to see that practice at first-hand, Hulme (1991).

[4] "The serious problems of life are never fully resolved. If ever they should appear to be so, it is a sure sign that something has been lost. The meaning and purpose of a problem seem to lie not in its solution, but in our working at it incessantly. This alone preserves us from stultification and petrification." (Bhaktin, cited in Hulme, 1991)

finds this more demanding as she goes deeper into the culture, relationships, and closer to the source of the tradition – Boston. This going deeper and testing her sense of reality and of her self is risk, jeopardy. This is part of the quest. What seems and what is get mixed up.

Boston: The reality at Boston University and the Massachusetts Mental Health Centre, as Annie found it, was monolithic, an institution in which abstraction (theory) was divorced from the specifics of situated practice. By contrast, Annie notes and relays the realities of the day-to-day life in the wards as she saw it, and as she interpreted it by being in relationship with those living it.

Annie found that her capacity to argue against the monolithic reality – to test it and to defend her self – was at risk. Partly this was due to a self-sealing epistemology in the dominant reality; in turn this was part of the more general problem that the 'reality' was constructed through the dominant interpretive schema. But Annie, the outsider, could see.

What can Annie - what can we - rely on then? From Annie's experience, we learn that if you are totally committed to this experience, or to participation, you can rely on *use of self.* Annie uses her experience of involvement with the patient – this fans the flames of her indignation, and it seems feeling is absolutely central to this experience – as indicating something other than what the dominant interpretive schema suggests. She uses her observation – of neglect, of the gap between what is professed and what is practised, of the self-sealingness of the epistemology of the schema and its effects.

But this is not sufficient – this alone might yield only dissonance and crisis. She needs another version of the dominant schema or (and/or) another schema to interpret these data from observation.

The difficulty with trying to interpret differently within the framework of the dominant schema (tradition), i.e. in Boston, or in the U.S. more generally, is that these data are not regarded as data. They don't get in as material which could challenge the schema (because they are already interpreted in its terms as evidence of something else, e.g. 'resistance'). MacIntyre notes a feature of epistemological crises:

'Until [the one facing a crisis] has adopted some schema he does not know what to count as evidence; until he knows what to treat as evidence he cannot tell what schema to adopt. Trapped in this epistemological circularity the general form of his problem is "what is going on here?"' (p. 243).

The value of reading and re-reading

We find that Annie, in the grip of an epistemological crisis, draws on two sources: *experience, informed by reading* and *re-reading.*

Annie draws on her experience of participation and involvement as a nurse; a nurse acting in the context of other relationships and in the context of another tradition and another community. This 'other' is the tradition of the therapeutic community, milieu therapy, and commitment to the principle of service to community. Annie acts and interprets, in her relationship with Mrs X, in the context of relationships with other patients.

Annie uses reading as one resource to reflect on and observe this. Literature provides a basis for seeing what others elsewhere have observed. She *uses* the schema from Boston. Greenblatt *et al* (1955), her Bible, on re-reading, still provides a schema, for interpretation: *now*, though, to *contrast* what she sees with what they said was there. She draws on another source – Koestler – to work out answers to painful questions: How does one come to believe (Annie's problem is construed in light of a more general problem of belief and disillusionment)? How does a belief system intertwine (with) power and language (again, the more general helps her understand her own experience)?

Resolutions: Drawing on these sources Annie moves towards

resolutions:

• within the terms of Boston tradition of the one-to-one relationship itself – in its own terms – the evidence is that the institution does not live up to its ideals (it is not coherent);

• in terms of the other tradition – that of service to community (or, to the individual in community) - the Massachusetts Mental Health Centre and BU School of Nursing fail. They are seen as a system linked to power, support of which is based on conversion. This system is epistemologically and ethically suspect.

We can get a sense of the significance of the within-tradition critique, by going back to Annie's 'bible'. I went back to this source, and noted a few pages from Greenblatt *et al* in which June Mellow's work, and the role of the nurse in that institution – the same institution in which Annie formed her relationship with Mrs. X – are described.

The text indicates that practice in Boston is progressive – it offers a different role for nurses (exemplar: June Mellow) and a schema for interpreting that practice. [But note: questions about the practice are relegated to a footnote.]

I noted, in a way I think I would not have done before, the reference to June Mellow and her work (Greenblatt *et al*, pp. 152-155). June Mellow is cast as an exemplar of both the 'extension of therapeutic functions to ward personnel' and "individual nursing therapy" with two patients, based on psychodynamic and therapeutic milieu principles. A claim was made by Greenblatt *et al* that, through the administrative and communication changes made to allow this form of therapy between Mellow as head nurse and the two patients, 'interest in all the patients was furthered and personnel were educated in a concrete experiential sense' (p. 154). We note that Greenblatt *et al* (1955) asked 'May we not conclude...that under proper conditions the traditional role of the psychiatric nurse can be augmented to include the function of individual therapist, a function heretofore almost exclusively reserved for the psychiatrist'.

This text implies that the one-to-one relationship represents a shift in 'tradition' in psychiatric nursing.

But it is in the footnote that we find Greenblatt *et al* attending to some further questions raised, in a footnote (p. 155). They say that the way psychiatric nurses' time may 'most profitably' be used is not yet determined; nor is the question of whether they should work with other staff, groups or individual patients:

'Intensive work with individual patients under the supervision of a psychiatrist perhaps seems like a wasteful extravagance when so many other patients are greatly in need of attention. This type of deep psychological experience, however, may be an essential step in helping nurses achieve sufficient understanding and insight into emotions *to enable them to move closer to all patients.*' (p. 155, emphasis added).

It seems, then, that Greenblatt *et al* were aware of the issues that concerned Annie in 1960-61. In particular, they were aware of the tension between individual therapy and concern for the group of patients, and the question of whose was the intended benefit of one-to-one therapy – patients, directly; or nurses, and perhaps then patients indirectly (through the nurse 'moving closer to all patients').

It seems Annie was addressing the issues Greenblatt *et al* note, on the basis of her observation that nurses, in practice, were not close to all patients. Was Annie herself trying to 'move closer to all patients' while also in the one-to-one relationship with Mrs. X? If so, this may be seen as enacting the values and principle of 'service to community' with attention to the one.

Annie, according to this reading, returns to questions *relegated or submerged* to a footnote in her 'bible'. I see that in doing so, she finds a basis for critique of the dominant tradition. She argues with it, and in doing so, partakes in that tradition. Through involvement in the setting, she finds the knowledge – bitter though it is. And in doing so, she upholds principles of the primordial ethic (Smith,

1982): charity and veracity (the best possible interpretation of that tradition).

MacIntyre writes that 'narrative requires an evaluative framework in which good or bad character helps to produce unfortunate or happy outcomes' (p 45). Annie is drawing attention to the 'degenerate' character of the tradition of the one-to-one relationship:

'it is a mark of a degenerate tradition that it has contrived a set of epistemological defenses that enable it to avoid being put in question or at least to avoid recognising that it is being put into question by rival traditions' (p. 250).

Return to the quest: Part of the quest story, then, is Annie's return to her source (Greenblatt *et al*) to bring back boons of argument (against a false image) and of relationship (to the community).

Annie's emotional response to the bitterness of finding this truth is worth noting. These resolutions are not – or not wholly – rational. Annie emphasizes the strength of her feelings when facing and trying to resolve this crisis. I read her texts as, in some sense, *a story of love betrayed.*

MacIntyre writes:

'For all persons who fall out of love and need to know how he or she can possibly be so mistaken...the relationship of seems to is becomes crucial...[this is the equivalent of the philosopher's] problem of justification of induction'. MacIntyre, pp. 241-242).

And Koestler - to whom Annie referred June Mellow, with advice to find there illumination of her feelings and response - wrote in *The God That Failed*:

"A faith is not acquired by reason. One does not fall in love with a woman, or enter the womb of a church, as a result of logical persuasion...A faith is not acquired; it grows like a tree. Its crown points to the sky; its roots grow downward into the past and are nourished by the dark sap of the ancestral humus." (Koestler, p. 25)

"I served the Community Party for seven years – the length of time Jacob tended Laban's sheep to win Rachel his daughter. When the time was up, the bride was led into his dark tent; only the next morning did he discover that his ardours had been spent not on the lovely Rachel but on the ugly Leah.

I wonder whether he ever recovered from the shock of having slept with an illusion. I wonder whether afterwards he believed that he had ever believed in it. I wonder whether the happy end of the legend will be repeated; for, at the price of another seven years of labour, Jacob was given Rachel, and the illusion became flesh. And the seven years seemed unto him but a few days, for the love he had for her." (Koestler, p 82)

These texts, then, document a phenomenon: *participation in* an epistemological crisis, reading, and particularly re-reading, enables Annie to observe the epistemological crisis from a point of critique within the tradition or from another tradition.

Reading helps Annie understand how she came to believe what she did in the first place (she read Greenblatt *et al*, related it to her own experiences, believed and followed). Reading helps her understand how what she believed in, and used as a good guide to reality, was wrong: it led to an epistemological crisis. It also led her into risk and peril (moral and epistemological).

Annie recovered from this peril by asking questions - in effect, by putting the tradition in question. At the centre of the *quest* is the *question*. For Annie the questions were: *Who is this for?* and *Whom do I serve?* The answers tell the quester what journey he or she is really on. This provides a better narrative, on the basis of which to proceed.

The better narrative, for Annie, is service to community, but with respect for the individual; not service to the individual (patient or nurse) at the expense of the community. [5] Annie knew this already – the answer is already present in the question. She knew because she had participated in that tradition before and knew it from experience (in her bones). [6] She knew from experience now how vulnerable it was, and how strong.

The boon, the good, of what Annie brought back was *not a split* of two traditions or narratives. She *holds the two in tension*: they are melded when told by her in her story. Annie is in relationship to both traditions, in telling a better story. That better story enables her to realise a good which might otherwise have been missed. (An example is her memory that Peplau's original practice was with a regressed patient with schizophrenia: what was good as nursing for that patient then become generalised, commodified, promulgated towards nurses forming one-to-one relationships with all sorts of

---

[5] I recall here my talk with Gus McLean, who said he has talked to a lot of ex-CP members. His line of thinking was:

Why did Communists recant in show trials? This was due to an ethic based on the power of the group or belief in the group; the belief that the good of the group is greater than the individual. Now we live in a society where ego is most important, so you can imagine the craziness this caused.

I link this to Annie: the power of the group at Boston University, they were not looking out, so it kept a kind of group think; thus a monolithic mentality. In terms of epistemology: what was emphasised in the monolithic thinking was the power of abstraction versus the particular (contra e.g. Martha Nussbaum's epistemology and ethics). Annie, however, noted the particulars of the situation, the ethnography: the story. For Annie, theory sounds OK – but doesn't fit reality. A question, then: Do we need realistic theory?

[6] See personal communication from Dr Tom Harrison. I told him about Annie's response of disillusionment about seeing the focus on one-to-one relationships and neglect of the rest of patients. He said that if you come from working in a therapeutic community to other places that do not have therapeutic community practices 'you can't understand how people can be so hoodwinked;' your response is 'beyond the rational;'; working in a therapeutic community, 'it gets into your bones about relationships, that you can't undo;' 'once you have crossed over the river…what it is back over the river – you can't understand their perceptions.'

other patients.)

For Annie, the stories in question are stories about what the good of psychiatric nursing is. The one-to-one relationship, or service to community? Or both?

Conclusion: the tradition of reading and re-reading texts in psychiatric nursing [7]

One other boon with which Annie returned was a quiver of questions from which she crafted the design of the study that became *Patient-Nurse Interaction* (Altschul, 1972):

'I shall have opportunity later to observe training through the one-to-one relationship. My observations so far leave me dubious of the value. It is my intention to see if patients here (in the UK) have similar experiences'.

The value of June Mellow's class was that she thought 'seriously about the way psychoanalytic concepts can be taught', which 'started a train of thought which I shall pursue for some time to come, namely to determine what really are the theoretical foundations on which psychiatric nursing is based'.

These questions, and Annie's responses – methodological and substantive – stimulated much further work and a significant line of UK psychiatric nursing research. [8]

Annie's texts demonstrate the value of reading when you need an

---

[7] My cycling thoughts of 15-11-01:
The quest thus becomes a theme. Annie went to get a boon, found her question, came back with boons or gifts of:
- Tradition shaped to her
- Argument against Boston University idol, and for knowledge needed
- Relationship: with USA and Boston University people, belonging, with Mrs. X.

[8] That line, though, took interaction rather than relationship as its central problem (see Tilley, 1997). Thirty years on we resume the conversation about relationship.

alternative tradition as guide to reality. They indicate the value of the quest, and its costs.

The texts are the product of, and show the value of, her method of doing participant observation, as ethnographer of the American scene, and in practice and supervision in Boston.

I hope that this reflection on Annie's texts from her visit to the U.S. in 1960-61 indicates the value of reading and re-reading – for Annie. I hope, too, that it indicates something about the value of reading in nursing. Reading helps us see the value of texts, writing, documenting. Through practice, writing, reading, and re-reading, we realise better the good of psychiatric nursing. We participate in a tradition shaped to - and by - writing, readings and re-readings of others. If I understand this, it is through re-reading Altschul, who re-read. Re-read, she still teaches us.

References

Greenblatt, M., York, R. H., and Brown, E. L. (1955) *From Custodial to the Therapeutic Patient Care in Mental Hospitals: Explorations in Social Treatment.* New York: Russell Sage Foundation.

Hulme, A. (1991) 'A comparative study of The Quest for Healing,' in Lindsay Clarke's *The Chymical Wedding*, and Naomi Mitchison's *The Corn King and the Spring Queen.* Unpublished MSc in General and Comparative Literature, University of Edinburgh.

Koestler, A. ***et al*** (1950) *The God That Failed: Six Studies in Communism.* London: Hamish Hamilton.

MacIntyre, A. (1985) *After virtue: a study in moral theory.* Guildford: Duckworth.

MacIntyre, A. F. (1989) 'Epistemological crises, dramatic narrative and the philosophy of science'. IN Clark SA and Simpson E (eds.) *Anti-theory in ethics and moral conservatism.* Albany: SUNY Press, pp. 241-261.

Smith, H. (1982) *Beyond the post-modern mind.* New York: Crossroad.

Tilley, S. (1999) 'Altschul's legacy in mediating British and American psychiatric nursing discourses: common sense and the 'absence' of the accountable practitioner'. *Journal of Psychiatric and Mental Health Nursing* 6 (4) 283-296.

Appendix 1

Re-Reading Altschul: Notes on Knowledge and Tradition

Stephen Tilley

Stephen Tilley PhD BA RMN; Senior Lecturer Nursing Studies; School of Health in Social Science; University of Edinburgh 31 Buccleuch Place, Edinburgh EH8 9JT, email: s.tilley@ed.ac.uk

'The practice of putting in question, whether within a tradition or between traditions, itself always requires the context of a tradition.' (Macintyre, p. 250)

Introduction

This paper was written for the *festschrift* held in November, 2001, to honour Annie Altschul's 'contributions to psychiatric nursing - past, present and future'. Annie was Professor Emeritus of Nursing Studies at The University of Edinburgh.[1] The paper was too long to give, and I gave a shorter and somewhat differently-focused paper (see Tilley 2003, 'Gifts of argument, relationship, and tradition: boons of re-reading Altschul'.)

But Annie said afterwards that she thought I should have given this paper. So I have re-drafted it, to bring out more clearly the original argument, and offer it here as an appendix to the works read on the day and Annie's own texts - such value as it may have depends on the context they provide.

I organised the *festschrift* around a set of papers Annie wrote about her 1960-61 visit to the United States and a set of responses to the papers. I was one of the respondents who used these papers as a stimulus to think and write about her contributions. I focused on the contribution Annie made to reading, and re-reading, psychiatric nursing literature. In her writings she conveyed her readings of others' writings, and the role of those readings on her 'quest for knowledge of mental illness' (Altschul, 1999) to inform her practice. But she did something more: she conveyed how her readings of texts outside the canon of psychiatric nursing literature (the example Koestler's *The God that Failed*) enabled her to resolve a crisis of knowledge. The crisis had been occasioned by her perception of a gap between the reality conveyed by the texts she read (the example what she called her 'bible', Greenblatt *et al*, 1955) and the reality she observed in practice. Finally, she conveyed the value of re-reading. Texts could play a role both in occasioning and in resolving an epistemological crisis. Annie thus contributed by documenting the role of reading and re-reading in working out questions arising from practice (of nursing and of teaching nursing) of the form '*What am I to do?*' and '*How could I have been so wrong?*' Such questions inevitably arise for practitioners and for the field itself, and an insight into how they arise and how they might be resolved constitutes a substantial contribution to psychiatric nursing practice and knowledge. Annie's work thus provided a valuable model, which I have tried to use in writing this paper. As Altschul read and re-read Greenblatt *et al* and Koestler, so I took the occasion of the *festschrift* to read and re-read Altschul.

In this paper I will present my reading of the set of *festschrift* papers, and indicate how it affects my reading and re-reading of Annie's later work, particularly her 1972 *Patient-Nurse Interaction* (PNI). Drawing on work by Alastair MacIntyre, I will argue that the 1960-61 texts shed light on a conflict of traditions; and that Annie appears, in the re-reading, as the central figure in this conflict. Annie experienced an epistemological crisis during her visit to the US and resolved it by challenging the dominant tradition and by constructing a narrative drawn from another tradition. That latter tradition of service to community - through practice, education and research - is one that I work to align myself with.

The example I have chosen is a significant one. I have argued elsewhere (Tilley, 1995; Tilley, 1999)[2] that PNI is a key text for understanding Annie's role in 'mediating' American and British psychiatric nursing discourses. The 'Introduction' to that text reviewed literature that Annie had read prior to going to the US, including Greenblatt *et al* (1955). It indicated the ways in which American texts had influenced her understanding of the importance of the patient-nurse relationship, and her framing of the problems and questions for the study which resulted in PNI. Her reading and re-reading played a key part in establishing a hermeneutic between American and British psychiatric nursing literature (and through that practice). I will outline how 1960-61 papers have occasioned my re-reading of PNI, and given me a different perspective on Annie's 'mediating' role.

While considering the value of re-reading Altschul in relation to a specific central text in British psychiatric nursing literature (PNI), I will also consider the value of re-reading more generally. Re-reading poses a challenge to the ideology currently dominant in psychiatric nursing literature, which focuses attention on use of the 'latest' (most recent) evidence as the basis for practice. Finally I will bring out the more general role of re-reading in resolving an epistemological crisis.

Annie's epistemological crisis in 1960-61

I will treat Annie's 1960-61 texts as sources for characterising and for understanding her epistemological crisis. I use Alasdair MacIntyre's (1989) notion of 'epistemological crisis' to mean the state one is in when what *is* conflicts with what *seems* - when one's way of knowing is put in question and one is forced to ask *How could I have been so wrong?* MacIntyre argues that to resolve such a crisis one needs a narrative of how one came to believe what one did in the first place, and a more inclusive narrative of how that was wrong. Those (needed) narratives, MacIntyre says, are grounded in traditions. I will describe how Annie's epistemological crisis arose from a conflict of traditions - the tradition of the one-to-one relationship and the tradition of the therapeutic community.

I will indicate how Annie resolved her epistemological crisis by putting in question the ideology of American nursing dominant at the time of her visit. The texts shed light more generally on Annie's practice of putting psychiatric nursing practice and education in question, and on the 'virtue' (MacIntyre, 1985) of putting in question itself.

First, what do I mean by 'putting in question'?

1. Annie put her own UK practice, prior to the trip, in question. She said that it did not provide an adequate basis for determining what to teach and how to teach during general nurses' short psychiatric experience. She also put her own practice in question when she said in the papers that she had practised and taught successfully without knowing the theoretical basis of psychiatric nursing.[3] It was against this background that she went to the US to answer some of these questions.

2. Once there she put in question the nursing practice she found. There were many good aspects. But there were noted problems - e.g. it was not based on an identifiable perspective; it was based on ideology; patients' perceptions and experience were not adequately considered.

3. Later, in research for her MSc degree aimed at answering questions stemming from her 1960-61 visit, and published as PNI (Altschul, 1972), she put Scottish psychiatric nursing in question.[4]

I will focus on two aspects of American psychiatric nursing practice and education which Annie put in question:

• She put lack of 'argument' into question - American (and later Scottish) nurses' apparent unwillingness to engage in argument; and the inadequacy of argument supporting the practice of one-to-one relationship

• She put the American tradition of the one-to-one relationship in question, by juxtaposing it to another tradition (grounded in her UK experience) - the tradition of service to community.

Finally, I will indicate three significant gifts - of argument, relationship, and tradition - which Annie bequeathed to us out of her crisis.

Narratives of Annie's Visit

To set the scene for this analysis, I will document my reading of Annie's 1960-61 texts as ethnographic narratives, or stories,[5] documents of the quest for knowledge which took her to the US.

1. 'The Report to Funders' - putting 'argument' in question.

Annie, faced with a practical problem of devising a curriculum for short placements for general nurses on psychiatric placements, and 'discontented with conditions as they were', had a principal aim: 'to find out how psychiatric nursing was incorporated into the basic comprehensive training course'. Having 'no idea' how to do this, she went to the US where she 'hoped to find clearly defined aims, well planned curricula and sound evaluation of psychiatric nursing experience'.

This initial problem, based on the initial motive, 'got least illumination'. The initial motive got displaced as Annie opened herself to new experiences, to friendships, and to the wider culture. The 'terms of reference' expanded to include the system of education, the structure of health care. Annie thought this necessary, as 'it is, of course, impossible to understand the significance of a people's attitude to work, to sickness and to the profession without a love of its culture'.[6] 'Love of culture' is a background epistemological resource for Annie, as the act changes to 'coming to belong'; the motive, to understand. Throughout, Annie notes the benefits and risks of moving from outsider to insider. In the course of her time in the US, her perspective had shifted - she was less critical of what she had known in Britain.

The story of the journey begun in California is thus: Annie goes out to find something out, finds out much more, loses sight of her aims but widens her perspective, and draws conclusions about a number of pertinent issues. These issues include: the value of comprehensive education, lack of clarity about what 'psychiatric experience can contribute', the 'disturbing' way in which 'students were introduced to psychiatric wards', the value of 'other nursing personnel', some limitations of 'nursing education in the U.S.A.'.

But she noted too that 'even the best organised life is meaningless for the patient. Very frequently nursing staff had conceptualised very well how hospital life was meant to help the patient but this was not experienced by the patient'. There was a gap between nurses' conceptualisation of what they were doing and the patient's experience. On the basis of this she set an intention.

She was able to make this observation because American nurses 'criticised themselves', 'did not avoid discussions in which shortcomings were discussed'. She noted the 'unembarrassed way Americans allowed (her) to see both what they thought good and what they thought bad'. Their doing so enabled her to observe and to compare practices.

But on the other hand, Annie noted 'few of the people I met are genuinely seeking knowledge for its own sake'; student nurses 'have not seen any nursing at all...they have no model at all and, therefore, no aim for themselves'.

Thus, by the end of her time in California, Annie was critical of the nurses' ability to account for their practice - though willing to discuss their work, they did not define the concepts they use, and do not examine the rationale for their practice; they did not explain aims, techniques, achievements. Their concentration on ward and group approaches was at the expense of knowledge of individual patients. She remarked on the loneliness of individual patients. Annie detected a disjunction between the dominant theory and the day-to-day management of patients.

Annie suspended judgement, tried to claim no more than was warranted by observation and interview, and set the agenda to test her forming views against experience:

'I shall have opportunity later to observe training through the one-to-one relationship. My observations so far leave me dubious of the value.'

2: Putting the one-to-one relationship in question.

'Later,' for Annie, was Boston, whence she went after California. It is in her account of Boston that the grounds for her general critique are most clearly laid out.

In her 'Report to Funders' on the whole visit to the US, Annie critiqued the emphasis, bias or imbalance in teaching of psychiatry in schools of nursing:

'There is a strong bias in all schools in the way psychiatry is presented and much of what is at best hypothetical is presented dogmatically as factual'.

This same imbalance is noted in relation to emphasis given to Peplau's work on the one-to-one relationship. The charges are dogmatism and idolatry: 'It was interesting to see the tremendous influence of Hildegard Peplau on all schools of nursing. Dr Peplau's book *Interpersonal Relations in Nursing* is treated with the reverence only the Bible deserves':

The film *Nurse-Patient Relationship* is shown everywhere...The special relationship - called everywhere a "ONE-to-ONE relationship"(sic)- is now considered to be the essence of psychiatric nursing and in many schools it is the only thing now being taught. In the extreme form, the student is told that during her period in the psychiatric ward her sole duty lies in finding one patient with whom to form a relationship.'

While Annie sees that this may benefit the student, helping the student learn about involvement and about 'entering into involvement without harm to herself', she was 'completely unable to find out how this is supposed to benefit the patient'. She does not think the ' "one-to-one relationship"...is the only thing that should be taught' and she is 'left wondering about its relevance to psychiatric nursing or to nursing in general'.

Annie criticises what she perceives as an uncritical, univocal, monolithic enterprise and technology of education based on Peplau's work and on the 'one-to-one relationship'; criticising it on the grounds of bias and undue reverence amounting to idolatry.

The Crisis - Doubts, Resistance, Protests and Principles

The texts as a whole document a serious breach with the one-to-one relationship tradition. Annie's suspicions had been raised in California, but the dramatic breach occurred in Boston, where an 'epistemological crisis' (MacIntyre, 1985) centred on a difference between what is and what seems: what Annie saw did not accord with reality as others around her perceived it.

The crisis was tied up with her sense of what she was doing on this journey. Her way of seeing and her experience seem to have shifted. She comments on how her writing was delayed by 'new experiences' that delayed her report. She says 'I no longer feel my aims have any relevance to my experience'. She had 'learning experiences so diverse' and 'satisfactions unrelated to my original purpose of enrolment [in Boston University School of Nursing]'.

We may say that the crisis occurred in Boston because it was here that Annie moved from observer to participant in a one-to-one relationship. It is here, too, that she emphasises most strongly the significance of relationships:

'Most valuable of all was, I think, the opportunity of having colleagues and of belonging...Everywhere else during my stay in the U.S.A. I was only a visitor'.

Part of the value of the experience lay in 'submerging in the ordinary life of the community'. We detect in that phrase the integrity of

Annie's method: she submerged herself in the life of American communities, especially Boston; and in the life of classrooms and wards in those communities, again especially in Boston. This is consonant with her view that love of the culture is necessary to understand the contexts of education, work, and relationships with the mentally ill.

The story is of Annie in Boston 'sufficiently involved...to see from the point of view', appreciative of the 'personal interest people have taken in me' to the extent that 'my memories of Boston University will remain permanently influenced by the personal relationships I have enjoyed', and 'belonging'.

In her report on Boston, Annie presents herself as in some way changed by her experience there. Her writing as participant observer, too, had changed. We hear her moving towards an insider position: she sees 'nursing problems in the USA from within rather than with reference to my own preoccupations'. She uses the term 'involvement' in describing this: 'At BU I was sufficiently involved to see nursing problems from the point of view of the student, the faculty...and the public.' 'Sufficient involvement' will become both means or method, of knowing, and setting for an epistemological crisis: participation in the everyday life as someone 'sufficiently involved' grants her a discomfiting but productive critical perspective.

In moving to this insider position she nonetheless did not give up her <u>principles</u>: she was 'unable to set aside even for a short period my rather firm conviction that *nursing is a service to the community*, and that students should learn to serve and to nurse' (italics added). While original aims might be lost, firm convictions were not.

Thus the plot of Annie's Boston narrative hinges on tension between two elements. On the one hand is a desire for and appreciation of belonging and submersion. On the other hand, Annie notes her own limits in being only 'sufficiently engaged', her inability to set aside the conviction of nursing as 'service to community', and the implied failure of her teachers to attend to obligations implied by 'students should learn to serve and to nurse'. An important element in the plot is that the culture, so open to belonging, is yet closed to argument, critique and self-perception. In the 'Miss Mellow' section she implies that the proffered tradition is not open to critique: 'I was also surprised that few of my colleagues appeared willing to defend their opinions if they were challenged, or seemed to enjoy pursuing an argument. This may have been due to their courtesy to me as a stranger, or they may have interpreted my enquiries as critical and may have acted defensively'.

Annie put the one-to-one relationship tradition in question in two ways. On the one hand, she resisted the practice. In the one-to-one relationship with Mrs X she resisted focusing on what Mrs X thought relevant, and in supervision with June Mellow, about this relationship, she resisted focusing on what June Mellow thought relevant. Instead, with each of these women, she situated the one-to-one relationship in the context of other relationships - accomplishing a kind of autodidactic meta-learning.

With Mrs X, the context she established as relevant was that of her own and Mrs X's relationships with other patients in the ward. Annie did so explicitly in her role of nurse. In doing so she enacted a tradition of nursing as service to community, seeing herself as learning to serve and to nurse, and holding herself accountable on that basis.

With June Mellow, the context was dual. Annie kept part of her relationship to self, to herself. She also kept the focus on her one-to-one relationship with Mrs X as construed in the context of Mrs X's and Annie's other relationships; rather than just the one-to-one relationship stripped of this context.[7]

By doing so, Annie faced conflicts. With Mrs X it was conflict over her role - Annie asserted herself as nurse not psychotherapist. With June Mellow it was conflict over interpretation of Annie's 'resistance'. June Mellow interpreted this in terms of Annie's problems of involvement. Annie does not deny such problems and acknowledges benefits of skilled supervision for addressing in part issues of relationship formation and loss. But for Annie the significant resistance is of another kind.

She resisted the one-to-one tradition, as she found it, in several ways. She resisted (participating in, enrollment in, socialisation into) the institutionalisation of knowledge in that tradition. Attention to limits of involvement is clear in Annie's comments on being a student in Miss Mellow's class. She noted that she was sometimes 'too much observer', and that if 'detached' she identified with the leader (Miss Mellow) and contributed nothing to the class.For example, she resisted the institutionalisation of knowledge by resisting presentation of hypothesis as truth in June Mellow's class:

'I cannot accept the belief that Freudian psychology is the only, or indeed the most important theoretical framework' and 'Even if it were, I have so far failed to see where in psychiatric nursing it is applied'.

The value of the class was that she thought 'seriously about the way psychoanalytic concepts can be taught', which 'started a train of thought which I shall pursue for some time to come, namely to determine what really are the theoretical foundations on which psychiatric nursing is based'.

The phrase 'started a train of thought' conveys the energy Annie brought to her work of thinking about practice in Boston, and its fruits. The phrase 'what really are' perhaps implies that psychoanalytic concepts were not the 'real' theoretical foundation of psychiatric nursing, or at least not the sole foundation.

Thus Annie refused to subject herself fully to the belief system, partly on the grounds that it is not the real basis of psychiatric nursing practice. She also refused to subject herself to it *completely*, in supervision with June Mellow.

I emphasise 'completely' because Annie participated in the one-to-one tradition to a point, but did not 'go native'. She retained her participant observer status. This enabled her both to see and to know the one-to-one tradition, but from the inside; and to see and to know it in relation to a wider sphere of relevance.

Though unpersuaded on the basis of her California experience about the benefit of the one-to-one relationship, Annie did not decline to form one in Boston. She accepted doing so as part of her experience as a student. What she did, though, was to resist the method of teaching and learning that was offered - i.e. the assignment to focus on choosing a patient and then on analysis of why she had chosen that patient. She thus resisted focusing on that prescribed framework for interpreting the meaning of the relationship. I presume that means she resisted making that analysis the focus of her supervision. Instead, she seems to have made her relationship-as-nurse with Mrs X the focus of her work with Mrs X; we do not know if she tried or succeeded in making that the focus of her supervision with Miss Mellow.[8] We might conclude that in doing so she enacted, or realised, a different version of the one-to-one relationship, a *questioning* version. I will return below to consider this more fully as indicating how Annie's methodological accountability differed from that of her U.S. colleagues.

Having formed a one-to-one relationship with Mrs X, Annie expressed doubts about its value in the context of a setting in which patients were treated generally in what she saw as a non-therapeutic environment and manner. She was angry and bitter about the discrepancy between what Greenblatt *et al*'s writing about the setting led her to expect and what she found.

Annie reflexively subjected her own perceptions and thinking to the same critical questioning she applied to others. She considered possible explanations - that she was depressed, or that her 'findings' or 'evidence' was biased by her limited involvement and 'resistance' (in the sense that psychoanalysts use the term). But she rejected these hypotheses or potential challenges to her views, citing contrary evidence or the inadequacy of the 'epistemological defense' of the psychodynamic tradition. In doing this reflexive thinking she uses an interpretive schema which I think derives from her main tradition, that of 'service to community'. I take it that that tradition considers behavior in terms of the person's relationships with a network of others, family, ward, etc., with the one-to-one relationship one among that network.

Re-Readings - Putting in question

One of the *practices* of putting something in question is re-reading. Re-reading does not reproduce the first reading, but instead situates it in a new horizon of understanding. It raises questions: what do we make of the text now, against a new backdrop of expectation, disillusionment, demand? The questions raised by Annie's re-reading concern the gap between theory and practice of the one-to-one relationship, interpretation of what is being done in Boston, and the implications of the monolithic institution.

Re-readings are an essential element in Annie's resolution of the 'epistemological crisis' she faced. I find support for this claim by relating her papers to a section of the book she says was her 'bible' until her faith in it was overthrown by experience on the U.S. trip: Greenblatt *et al*'s (1955) *From Custodial to Therapeutic Care in Mental Hospitals*. In effect she deconstructed the one-to-one tradition by bringing out contradictions in, contradictions I have claimed are subjugated in (a footnote in) that 'bible'. She does this in part by citing the authority of a text from that tradition, Koestler's *The God That Failed*; referring her supervisor, exemplar and propagator of the one-to-one relation, to that text.

In short, Annie resisted - to an extent - the practices of truth production. This was interpreted by the supervisor as 'resistance' to the experience by which truth can be known. She resisted 'conversion'. She also identified, I think, one of the mechanisms which might have effected conversion. The counterpart to the self-protecting ideology was insularity, another form of defense against potentially disconfirmatory information. Annie says: 'Throughout my stay I was conscious of local colour influencing my thinking. Not until I left did I become aware of the extent of this influence...The predominance of local references in bibliographies was one aspect of this that struck me forcefully. The more subtle implications escaped me until after I had left Boston.'

In the 'Field Study' section Annie notes the value of seeing the hospital from the patients' point of view. She sees value, for the student, in the one-to-one relationship: 'This method of teaching helps the student to understand and cope with emotional involvement', provided there is good supervision. However she 'remained entirely unconvinced of the value of relationship therapy or nursing therapy, to the patient - in fact it seems patently unfair that students should use patients to learn about their own psychopathology.'

Annie also anticipates (in the manner of the good arguer) 'objections' to her views on the one-to-one relationship. Her objections could be countered 'by pointing to the fact that I remained detached and used defences against greater emotional involvement. Had I experienced more fully the impact of involvement I might have become more convinced of its value.'

But Annie challenges this challenge to the warrant for her original claims. She challenges the warrant for the counter challenge:

'This kind of argument would render nursing therapy as invulnerable and as immune to criticism as psychoanalysis is already. If only the initiated and converted are entitled to discuss, and only to praise and not to criticise, one cannot wonder at onlookers who dismiss the subject as unscientific. As a partial onlooker I remain doubtful.'

In the end, Annie adopted a position - indeed, it seems, the only possible position - from which to form a view of the practice of one-to-one relationship: in between believer and sceptic, belonging and remaining 'detached'. But it is exactly this pain of mediation that seems problematic. For the crisis seems to relate both to her unhappiness and bitterness at the loss of what she wanted to believe in; and to her dissatisfaction with an inauthentic version of what she had believed in. She - as a scientist - cannot believe in what is offered to her because it does not accord with reality. That gift is rejected: It is an illusion. The problem she then faces is *how she could have been so illusioned.* It is in her attempt to answer this question that she re-reads her 'bible'. And what she gets is the boon of knowledge.

Annie's narrative of disillusionment is a problem of this kind. The reader senses that, if she was not in some sense 'in love' with the notion of the 'one-to-one relationship', her account of Greenblatt *et al* (1955) as her 'bible' and her emphasis that hers were 'big feelings' indicate that she nonetheless faced an epistemological crisis of some importance. She was 'illusioned' by this text.

In Annie's case, how she could have been so 'illusioned'? She blames the image-making writing, and counsels "don't write" (create a graven image).

Becoming disillusioned entailed being subject to 'radical interpretive doubts'; being faced with two competing 'schema of interpretation':

'Until [the one facing a crisis] has adopted some schema he does not know what to count as evidence; until he knows what to treat as evidence he cannot tell what schema to adopt. Trapped in this epistemological circularity the general form of his problem is "what is going on here?' (MacIntyre, 1989, p. 243).

This insight is pertinent to Annie's comments on June Mellow, in Annie's feedback report.

MacIntyre writes: 'Narrative requires an evaluative framework in which good or bad character helps to produce unfortunate or happy outcomes' (p 45). Annie calls into question the 'character' of the one-to-one tradition. I read her as drawing attention to the 'degenerate' character of the tradition of the one-to-one relationship, in the sense that MacIntyre used this notion:

'It is a mark to a degenerate tradition that it has contrived a set of epistemological defenses that enable it to avoid being put in question or at least to avoid recognising that it is being put into question by rival traditions' (p. 250).

This seems an apt characterisation of the situation Annie found herself in. She was faced with the kind of problem Alasdair Macintyre describes in a text entitled: 'Epistemological crises, dramatic narrative and the philosophy'. He cites similarities between problems 'ordinary agents' face and those considered by philosophers: 'For all persons who fall out of love and need to know how he or she can possibly be so mistaken...the relationship of *seems* to *is* becomes crucial...[this is the equivalent of the philosopher's] problem of justification of induction'. (pp. 241-242).

Annie refers June Mellow to Arthur Koestler (1950) but provides no page references or quotations. Reading Koestler I found the following:

"A faith is not acquired by reason. One does not fall in love with a woman, or enter the womb of a church, as a result of logical persuasion...A faith is not acquired; it grows like a tree. Its crown points to the sky; its roots grow downward into the past and are nourished by the dark sap of the ancestral humus."(p. 25)

"As a rule, our memory romanticized the past. But when one has renounced a creed or been betrayed by a friend, the opposite mechanism sets to work. In the light of that later knowledge, the original experience loses its innocence, becomes tainted and rancid in recollection. I have tried in these pages to recapture the mood in which the experiences related were originally lived - and know that I have failed."(pp 63-4)

"I served the Community Party for seven years - the length of time Jacob tended Laban's sheep to win Rachel his daughter. When the time was up, the bride was led into his dark tent; only the next morning did he discover that his ardours had been spent not on the lovely Rachel but on the ugly Leah.

I wonder whether he ever recovered from the shock of having slept with an illusion. I wonder whether afterwards he believed that he had ever believed in it. I wonder whether the happy end of the legend will be repeated; for, at the price of another seven years of labour, Jacob was given Rachel, and the illusion became flesh. And the seven years seemed unto him but a few days, for the love he had for her."(p 82)

We can read or re-read other texts in light of Annie's 1960-61 texts.

I looked at Greenblatt *et al* (1955) and noted - in a way I think I would not have done before, the reference to June Mellow and her work (pp. 152-155). June Mellow is cast as an exemplar of both the 'extension of therapeutic functions to ward personnel' and of 'individual nursing therapy" with two patients, based on psychodynamic and therapeutic milieu principles. A claim was made that through the administrative and communication changes made to allow this form of therapy between Mellow as head nurse and the two patients 'interest in all the patients was furthered and personnel were educated in a concrete experiential sense' (p. 154). We note that Greenblatt *et al* (1955) asked 'May we not conclude...that under proper conditions the traditional role of the psychiatric nurse can be augmented to include the function of individual therapist, a function heretofore almost exclusively reserved for the psychiatrist'. This implies that the one-to-one relationship represents a shift in 'tradition' in psychiatric nursing. Greenblatt *et al* attend to some questions raised, in a footnote (p. 155), noting that the way psychiatric nurses' time may 'most profitably' be used is not yet determined; nor is the question of whether they should work with other staff, groups or individual patients:

'Intensive work with individual patients under the supervision of a psychiatrist perhaps seems like a wasteful extravagance when so many other patients are greatly in need of attention. This type of deep psychological experience, however, may be an essential step in helping nurses achieve sufficient understanding and insight into emotions to enable them to move closer to all patients.' (p. 155).

This suggests that Greenblatt *et al* were aware of the issues which concerned Annie in 1960-61 - particularly the tension between individual therapy and concern for the group of patients, and the question of whose was the intended benefit of one-to-one therapy - patients, directly, or nurses, and perhaps then patients indirectly (through the nurse 'moving closer to all patients'). Indeed, they could be seen as motivated by a concern for and affinity with (or closeness to) 'all patients'.

It seems Annie was addressing the issues Greenblatt *et al* note, and that her observation was that nurses, in practice, were not close to all patients. Annie herself tried to 'move closer to all patients' while also in the one-to-one relationship with Mrs X. This may be seen as enacting the values and principle of 'service to community' with attention to the one.

We note, too, precursors of continuing concern over nurses' time and attention to individuals, with the risk of failure to attend to others 'greatly in need of attention' (Gournay and Brooking, 1994; Tilley and Ryan, 2000).

The Gifts of Putting Into Question

The fruits of Annie's putting into question are:

• the gift of argument (through argument about argument, toward a notion of the better argument)

• the gift of relationship (through argument about relationships, towards a notion of the better relationship)

• the gift of tradition (through argument about traditions, towards a notion of the better tradition)

The notion of the 'better' here is grounded in the practices and principles Annie exemplifies and models in the texts. The principal gift is the tradition of relationship with those with whom we can argue about the good of psychiatric nursing.

The gift of argument

Annie's main method of argument in these papers is making claims based on participant observation. The warrant for many of the claims she makes is that she knows because she took part in a social process, using her self to reflect on it.[9]

'Argument' as content is also a theme in the papers. She notes that nurses in some settings opened up their work, good and bad, to scrutiny; but also that they generally did not question it (with qualifications - research, for example, is being taught). This lack of argument contrasts with her practice and values.

She provides the grounds for an argument about the kind of further inquiry or research which is needed. This forms the basis for the methodology she developed for her MSc study. In that study she asked nurses to account for what they did in interaction which she had observed. She argued, in her analysis, about the validity of their accounts.

The gift of relationship

Annie's visit was rich in relationships - with colleagues, patients, the public, the American people and society. These relationships, her reflexive relationship with herself, are the backdrop to and the data from her participant observation. Themes of moving from stranger to belonging, and of involvement, run through the texts.

In the texts, argument is always seen, or heard, in the context of relationship. Mrs. X the patient argues with Annie in the context of the one-to-one relationship. Annie argues with June Mellow in the context of the supervision relationship. Annie puts the issue of relationship in question, in the context of her relationships with Mrs. X and with June Mellow, and more generally with patients and nurses with whom she had relationships. She does so in the context of the teacher-reader or teacher-student relationship. Annie's role in these relationships is nurse teacher learning what to teach.

The gift of tradition

Annie sets the one-to-one relationship (the one she formed with Mrs. X, and more generally) in the context of these other relationships with patients. She links this to a moral context of obligation to 'community'.

These two traditions - that of the one-to-one relationship, and that of obligation and service to community - are in conflict, in Annie's experience. This conflict is the scene of the epistemological crisis.

By setting the one-to-one relationship in the context of relationships the nurse and patient have with others, Annie the nurse (as participant observer) sees the limits of arguments based on a more restricted gaze.[10]

Boston University School of Nursing held the one-to-one relationship to be the centre of psychiatric nursing. In the context of relationships with colleagues there and in the context of relationships with patients at Massachusetts Mental Health Centre, Annie argued against the uncritical promotion of this version of psychiatric nursing as the sole version.

What may have begun with the personal influence of key figures - Hildegard Peplau at Rutgers, perhaps Anne Hargreaves and June Mellow in Boston - had become a school, and a technology, powerful in shaping student nurses' relationships, and the sense of what psychiatric nursing was as a discipline. In other words, it had been institutionalised. This institutionalisation, and its associated discursive activities, are what I mean by the one-to-one relationship tradition. Annie came to the US influenced by writings in this tradition, especially her 'Bible' (Greenblatt *et al*, 1955).

But she came too from another tradition - that of Mill Hill, early therapeutic community work, milieu therapy. I take it that any one relationship in these environments was seen in the context of other relationships, and that these relationships were open to or subjected to a different kind of observation and question than in the one-to-one tradition. This tradition, grounded in the therapeutic community tradition, we can call the tradition of 'service to community'.[11]

In these papers, then, we see Annie mediating and articulating an argument about the relationship between two traditions: that of the one-to-one relationship and that of service to community. The boons of the quest she undertook underpinned part of her project for UK-based research - 'It is my intention to see if patients here (in the UK) have similar experiences [to those in the US]' - and the study born of that intention, published as *Patient-Nurse Interaction* (Altschul, 1972). The texts of subsequent psychiatric nursing research in the UK often suggest the insights, and disquiet, gained by readers and re-re-readers of her work. They constitute in textual form a (still live) line sustaining relationship and tradition.

Conclusion: Return to epigraph

'The practice of putting in question, whether within a tradition or between traditions, itself always requires the context of a tradition.' (Macintyre, p. 250)

In conclusion, I am claiming Annie as a source for a tradition to which I would like to claim allegiance: the tradition of those who put things in question. A nurse who does this can claim kinship with philosophers and scientists, among others. But there is a peculiar twist for mental health nurses. For they often, in their day to day practice, draw on common sense, make it a topic and use it as a resource in argument with 'mad' people. The 'mad' may put in question the common sense of the community, or challenge people to ask 'What is going on here?' But the social construction of reality theorists and the ethnomethodologists (e.g. Schultz, Berger and Luckmann, and Garfinkel) have taught us that it is risky to put common sense into question: we do so only at the risk of shaking the foundations of our sense of reality and the basis of our everyday cooperative interaction. Annie's experience raised questions for her, and she raises questions for us, about the boundaries of the common sense of the wider community, the group to which the individuals in one-to-one relationships belong, and the common sense of the nurses subscribing to the ideology of the one-to-one relationship. In putting the latter tradition into question Annie was affirming an older (in her experience) epistemology, grounded both in more radical questioning and in the sense generated through talk and argument in community. The tradition I claim through here is the one whose conversation is informed by that epistemology.

The allusions above to 'love', and the Koestler quotations, may seem obscure. What has love to do with Annie's experience and response? I think - feel - that the content, and tone, of her report on Boston, and especially her reference to Koestler, point in this direction. The Bible is not only an authoritative text. It is also a symbol of deep affiliation and covenant (viz. 'people of the Book'). We infer that Annie saw American nurses' regarding or treating Peplau's *Interpersonal Relations in Nursing* as misplaced; yet Annie referred to Greenblatt et al. as her 'bible'.

I believe that something akin to love is at the heart of Annie's response to her Boston experience. John Macmurray (1957, p. 15) summarised his philosophical position: 'all meaningful knowledge is for the sake of action, and all meaningful action is for the sake of friendship.' Macmurray was Professor of Moral Philosophy at the University of Edinburgh and as Dean of the Faculty of Arts was instrumental in bringing the then Nursing Studies Unit into that Faculty (Costello, pp. 336-337). He described himself as 'godfather' to what became the Department of Nursing Studies, which Annie joined in 1964. I think that Annie would have seen his philosophical position as akin to hers.

The matters of thought and argument that I have been teasing out in this paper are meaningful insofar as they inform action. Annie's impulse to new experience and thought about that experience was motivated by a desire to change and develop practice (action) in relation to people suffering mental distress ('compassionate'; see footnote viii). And that action was motivated by 'affinity'. Huston Smith (1982) suggested that motivation begets epistemology, which begets ontology, which begets anthropology. Annie's motivation of friendship and communion begot her epistemology. That far I can go. And that affinity is what I mean here by 'love'. Annie's anticipation of affinity with June Mellow's practice was shaken, occasioning epistemological crisis. My affinity with Annie sparks my own quest to tease out the epistemological issues in our relationship.

How could I have been wrong about Annie's argument in *Patient-Nurse Interaction*? Because I failed to see the sense of relationship that informed the arguments. This is akin to failing to see the sense of relationship that lies behind everyday, commonsense practices, Annie's variant of the solution to the problem of intersubjectivity which Harre detected in Schutz's work (Harre, 1983). Perhaps it is to mental health nurses in Annie's tradition that we should look for everyday heroic (heroine-ic) solutions to the particular problems of intersubjectivity entailed by affinity with and participation in community with those suffering mental disorders.

In summary, what did Annie's visit achieve? Peter Nolan, one of the respondents to the *festschrift*, thinks it was:

'a turning point in British (psychiatric) nursing', in that it heralded the importance of having a theoretical and literature bases for nursing. Her report coincided with the initiation of integrated training, where general nurses and psychiatric nurses spent a period of three months in each other's environments with the aim of acquiring relationship skills by interacting with patients. The emphasis on interpersonal relationships can be traced also to this time and it is highly likely that her report was instrumental in bringing this about. At this time also we see the inclusion of psychology and sociology into the nursing curricula coupled with the importance of seeing patients in their social contexts.' (Nolan, personal communication)

I see the following conclusions from Annie's visit as relevant to psychiatric and mental health nursing today. There was much to value in American psychiatric nursing practice, but some of the best work was done not by nurses but by psychiatric technicians. The value of learning nursing in a higher education institution was not fully realised, insofar as students did not question the authority of teachers and texts. American nurses were ready to open up their practice and talk about it to a stranger, but there was a gap between the practice they described and what Annie saw and experienced. The tradition of nursing as service was not valued. Nurses whose work with patients was framed by the ideology of the one-to-one relationship, in the form practised in Boston, and in the form promoted in Peplau's work, did not evidently attend to the institutionally-structured and institutionally determined social dimensions of patients' experience in hospital - at a cost to the patients.

Peter Nolan highlights the following issues in Annie's 1960-61 papers, as significant for the subsequent development of British psychiatric nursing:

• the importance of cross-cultural comparisons in nursing - Annie Altschul was one of the first to do that.

• the importance of getting outside one's context - this was included in some curricula subsequently as overseas placement.

• the inportance of spending time with mentors - with implications for clinical supervision, etc..

• the importance of developing observational skills and how to prepare students to use these.

• the importance of keeping field notes and writing one's experiences - very little of that is done now in training.

• the importance of being able to analayse texts - she also wanted to put psychiatric nursing on a stronger academic footing. (Nolan, personal communication)

I would point to three ways in which Annie's visit influenced subsequent British psychiatric nursing. Firstly, Annie's mixture of respect for some aspects of American culture and nursing practice, and disillusionment with the dominant forms of American psychiatric nursing, provided a new and different point of departure for British psychiatric nurses developing their practice and research. Secondly, Annie's integration of practitioner and researcher roles, in participant observation entailing use of self and development of relationships informed by the virtues of 'commitment to those suffering from mental distress,...affinity with them, and quest for knowledge about mental illness' provided an epistemological model which continues to influence British psychiatric mental health and psychiatric nursing practice.

Annie's visit bequeathed something else, profoundly relevant to today's practice and research. She raised the question of accountability mediated by text, subverting any easy certainty with her 'don't publish' admonition. In two connected texts - the *Report on the one-to-one Relationship with Mrs X, Boston* and her *Feedback to Supervisor June Mellow on the one-to-one relationship* - she both fulfils requirements of accountability in practice and education and then, speaking up to authority, questions the basis of those requirements. Forty years later, how are we to do this in today's evidence-based, protocol-guided, meta-analysis-biased world?

Annie's texts and her work overall provide not only a wide range of resources for reading and re-reading, but a set of motives for doing so. We can read to see into and understand a different way of life relevant to nursing, to feed imagination of possibilities 'elsewhere' (and risk disillusionment), to learn to relate our 'little' struggles in nursing to 'great' struggles in other social and political domains (and ourselves as nurses to ourselves as social and political beings). We have been left a legacy of asking to what and to whom do our words and our readings commit us? On whose words do we depend in determining how to proceed in interaction, relationship and community? Annie teaches that if we embark (or are cast) upon a quest such as hers, a quest in 'real' time and space and in dimensions opened by reading and re-reading, we will learn, but at the cost of epistemological crisis, and return less illusioned.

References

Altschul, A. (1972b) *Study of the multi-disciplinary approach to psychiatric treatment provided by Dingleton Hospital in the Border counties.* Dingleton Hospital: Melrose.

Altschul, A. (1972a) *Patient-Nurse Interaction*, Churchill Livingstone, Edinburgh.

Altschul, A. (1983) *The effectiveness of the Community Psychiatric Services provided by Dingleton Hospital for psychogeriatric patients in the Borders.* Scottish Office Home and Health Department: Edinburgh.

Altschul, A. (1999) Note written by Altschul, accompanying the photo presented to her, in the Department of Nursing Studies, University of Edinburgh, to celebrate her 80th birthday.

Blum, A. & McHugh, P. (1985) *Self-Reflection in the Arts and Sciences.* Humanities Press Atlantic Highlands, New Jersey.

Costello, J.E. (2002) *John Macmurray: A biography.* Floris: Edinburgh.

Greenblatt, M., York, R.H., and Brown, E.L. (1955) *From Custodial to the Therapeutic Patient Care in Mental Hospitals: Explorations in Social Treatment.* Russell Sage Foundation: New York.

Harre, R. (1983) *Personal Being.* Oxford: Basil Blackwell.

Hulme, A. (1991) 'A comparative study of The Quest for Healing', in Lindsay Clarke's *The Chymical Wedding*, and Naomi Mitchison's

The Corn King and the Spring Queen. Unpublished M.Sc. in General and Comparative Literature, University of Edinburgh.

Koestler, A. et al. (1950) *The God that Failed - Six Studies in Communism.* London: Hamish Hamilton.

MacIntyre, A. (1985) *After virtue: a study in moral theory.* Duckworth: Guidlford.

MacIntyre, A.F. (1989) 'Epistemological crises, dramatic narrative and the philosophy of science'. IN Clark SA and Simpson E (eds.) *Anti-theory in ethics and moral conservatism.* SUNY Press: Albany, pp. 241-261.

MacMurray, J. (1957) *The self as agent.* London: Faber and Faberl.

Peplau, H. (1952) *Interpersonal relations in nursing.* New York: GP Putnam's Sons.

Smith, H. (1982) *Beyond the post-modern mind.* New York: Crossroads.

Szasz, T. (1979) *The myth of psychotherapy: Mental healing as religion, rhetoric and repression.* Oxford: Oxford University Press.

Tilley, S. (1995) *Negotiating realities.* Avebury, Aldershot.

Tilley, S. (2002) A note on Annie Altschul, Emeritus Professor of Nursing Studies, The University of Edinburgh. *Journal of Psychiatric and Mental Health Nursing.* 9 (2) 128-130.

Tilley, S. (1999) Altschul's legacy in mediating British and American psychiatric nursing discourses: common sense and the 'absence' of the accountable practitioner. *Journal of Psychiatric and Mental Health Nursing.* 6 (4) 283-296.

Footnotes

[1] Annie died on 24th December 2001.

[2] On reading AA 1960/61 I re-read Patient-Nurse Interaction (PNI) (Altschul, 1972) I saw it as, and critiqued it as, a study of interaction in the first instance, and only secondarily about relationship. That reading was justified, I think. But now I see it more clearly as arising out of her continuing engagement in an argument about the one-to-one relationship - its value and its status as the basis of psychiatric nurses' practice. And seeing it thus, I see PNI as related to the tradition in which the one-to-one relationship is regarded as the core of psychiatric nursing; but as articulating a different tradition based on 'service to community'. I have argued elsewhere (Tilley, 1999) that the main legacy of PNI was a body of subsequent research on British psychiatric nursing, focusing on issues of interaction and the problem of nurses' accountability for their practice. Annie's 1960/61 papers are a resource for understanding anew her *Patient-Nurse Interaction* (1972) that I have elsewhere characterised (Tilley, 1999) as a pivotal text in British psychiatric nursing literature. It is central in that it provided a key reference point for subsequent work - including that by Cormack, MacIlwaine, etc. Its is central too because it frames a key problem: the psychiatric nurse's accountability. It method of observation and interviews to get accounts of practice, was used by others subsequently to study psychiatric patient-nurse interaction and clarify the role of the nurse. A number of subsequent writers have taken up Annie's finding that psychiatric nurses did not practice on the basis of an identifiable perspective. Generally this is seen as problematic, as it limits accountability (the accountable nurse seems to be absent, not present) and the potential for incremental practice development. But reading Altschul's 60/61 papers and re-reading PNI, I construe more clearly the place of Annie's work in relation to another stream or thread - work on psychiatric nurses in the community. AA 60/61 sensitises me to the values base of Annie's work, and to her 'interpretive schema'. Annie is part of the one-to-one relationship tradition, insofar as she engages in argument about what it means to be part of that tradition; and part of the person-in-community tradition.

[3] This raised questions: Does practice depend on theory? What does 'successful' mean in this context?

[4] My PhD thesis (published as Tilley, 1995) was in part an attempt to challenge the basis on which she put the Scottish practice in question. She found that nurses gave accounts of their interaction with patients in which they seemed to think that the reason they had done what they had done was self-evident; that it was 'common sense'. Annie thought it not obviously common sense, particularly as different nurses did different things in what Annie saw as the same situation.

[5] The story as I see it is a version of the quest story. Here I draw on Andrea Hulme's (1991) account of aspects of the quest. 'The main protagonist, quester or hero undertakes a journey which is realised on both an external, physical level and in terms of inner reflectiveness.' We can see the first part of this in terms of Annie's external visit, her travels, to and in the US, and the activities she undertook including the one-to-one relationship. The second part is in the sense of her mind, and her feelings, we get through her reflexive account of the travel and its meaning for her. The quest has three stages: 1) starting out, 2) the ordeals leading to the acquisition of the reward; 3) return: 'The first of the quest stages begins with an initial separation of the main quester from his/her accustomed reality...The quest is initiated by some kind of radical or painful split in their world which heralds a change in their once stable relationship with their surroundings.' (Hulme, 1991) For Annie, the change was associated with the need to teach a different group of nurses in a different way. This was one change in stable relationships with her surroundings. Another was the change from her UK setting of practice. Another was the change from reading about a different kind of practice - the image of psychiatric and psychiatric nursing practice she had from Greenblatt *et al* (1995) - to observing, and participating in, that practice at first-hand.

[6] In this we hear precursors to her note accompanying a portrait of herself, commissioned by the Department of Nursing Studies, The University of Edinburgh. Annie wrote: 'My passionate concern for people who suffer from mental disorder, my affinity with them and my quest for knowledge about mental illness have never flagged.' Annie chose to sit for the portrait with a painting in the background, a rural scene brought by Annie's mother 'when she joined me in exile'. This symbolises Annie's grounding of her sense of self as person and professional in her culture, her cultures.

[7] We might indeed ask whether Annie ever did form a one-to-one relationship with Mrs X in the sense the Boston University School of Nursing construed that relationship. The theoretical question would be whether Annie and Mrs X were 'ones' in their relationship, as Annie construed and participated in it.

[8] We may say that in doing so Annie resisted the truth-producing practices of the school of one-to-one relationship nursing. She did so, we know, on ethical grounds. And we can see that this ethical decision is one phase of an ethical-epistemological act. Having chosen to act as she did on principle, she could not know in some ways, and could know in others.

Another way of saying this is to say that she was methodologically accountable within her tradition, and within her intended story or account-relationship with Mrs X (acting in the relationship so as to be able to tell a story about the relationship) and in her intended story or account-relationship with June Mellow (acting in her relationship with Mrs X and in her relationship with June Mellow so as to be able to tell a story about the relationship). She was able to provide a narrative about how she came to believe that one way of acting was good (realised a principle), how she came to realise that it was not (conflicted with her principle), and how she realised the principle in light of which it was not good.

She returned to sources: to texts - Greenblatt *et al* (1955) and Koestler (1950). Returning to Greenblatt *et al* (1955) helped her see the discrepancy between the 'is' represented there and the 'is' she saw in Massachusetts Mental Health Centre. She realises that the former 'is' is a 'seems'. But how to account for that - for having mistaken a 'seems' for an 'is'? This is the problem MacIntyre considers, and Koestler. There are different possible answers: she took the text to be true, i.e. to correspond to the reality of practice, and it was not (perhaps Greenblatt *et al* misled her); she took the text, which was true, to correspond to the current reality and it did not (the error was hers - expecting or assuming that a representation at one point in time would be valid at another); she took the text to be true, and the text was represented as being true still, and it was not (the error is due to those who claimed the text was still true, when it was not; perhaps colleagues at Boston University).

The standards Annie expresses or enacts are dual: epistemological (a standard of epistemological and scientific integrity; science as the way to truth); and ethical (service to the community). We can say, then, that Annie set her own standards for her comportment in the relationship with Mrs X and in her relationship with June Mellow. In acting in light of those standards, she clarified the standard - this a kind of self-reflection (Blum and McHugh, 1985). The standard is grounded in her notion of nursing - as service to community.

I found further insights into these issues in personal communication with Dr. Tom Harrison. I told him about Annie's response of disillusionment about seeing the focus on one-to-one and neglect of the rest of patients. He said if you go from working in a therapeutic community to work in other places 'you can't understand how people can be so hoodwinked'. Your response is 'beyond the rational'. Working in a therapeutic community 'it gets into your bones about relationships, that you can't undo'. Once you have 'crossed over the river', 'what it is back over the river - you can't understand their perceptions'. I heard him talking about an epistemological crisis summed up in 'you can't understand how people can be so hoodwinked'. Or in Annie's case, how she could have been so 'illusioned'. This is a counterpart to Koestler's narrative of illusion and disillusionment.

Annie blames the image-making writing for, in effect, creating a graven image. Annie's narrative of disillusionment is indeed like Koestler's. The reader senses that, if not 'in love' with the notion of the 'one-to-one relationship', her account of Greenblatt *et al* (1955) as her 'bible', and her emphasis that hers were 'big feelings', indicate that she faced an epistemological crisis of some importance. She had 'radical interpretive doubts', and faced the problem of two competing 'schema of interpretation': 'Until [the one facing a crisis] has adopted some schema he does not know what to count as evidence; until he knows what to treat as evidence he cannot tell what schema to adopt. Trapped in this epistemological circularity the general form of his problem is "what is going on here?' (p. 243). - this is pertinent to Annie and June Mellow, in Annie's feedback.

[9] Throughout the texts she presents little arguments - claims made on the basis of evidence of what she has seen or been told, supported by the warrant of first-hand observation and reflection, with appropriate qualifications. In doing so she evinces the hallmarks of the good rhetorician:

As the base rhetorician uses language to increase his own power, to produce converts to his own cause, and to create loyal followers to his own person, so the noble rhetorician uses language to wean men from their inclination to depend on authority, to encourage them to think and speak clearly, and to teach them to be their own masters... (Weaver, cited in Szasz, 1979, p 20)

She evinces too the values of the primordial ethic (Huston Smith, 1982: evincing the virtues of charity - seeing the other as fully one; humility, seeing one as equal to the other; and veracity, seeing both as they truly are).

[10] We can see this theme in Annie's later work on changes in practices when Dingleton Hospital psychiatric nurses moved into the community.

[11] For example, Annie, in research done at Dingleton Hospital in Scotland (Altschul, 1972b, 1983), described the practices in the in-patient therapeutic community at that hospital including talk among staff about their varying interpretations of the 'same' interaction. The practice in those wards was shaped by those conversations. When Dingleton nurses began working on their own in the community, they lost the basis for that kind of practice, because no-one else saw or could interpret what they did with the patient.

Appendix 2

Attendance and apologies

Present at the Festschrift	Apologies

Margaret Alexander
Crispin Allen
Annie Altschul
Phil Barker
Deborah Gibbons
David Glenister
Christine Howden
Maggie Ip
Mathew Lupton
Helen MacKinnon
Jessica MacLaren
Susan McGann
Barbara Mortimer
Peter Nolan
Bill Reynolds
Sue Robertson
Nancy Roper
Desmond Ryan
Alison Shankland
Val Sharkey
Neville Singh
Susan Sladden
Stephen Tilley
Rosemary Weir
Margaret Auld
Halla Beloff
Joy Bray
Kathleen Fraser
Melissa Hardie
Lisbeth Hockey
Danny Kelly
Noel Kreitman
Win Logan Gordon
Ian MacMillan
Peggy Nuttall
Robert Samuel
Ruth Schrock
Henry Walton
Sarah Whitcher

Bibliography of the works and publications of Professor Annie Altschul

Based upon the holdings of the Royal College of Nursing Archives Collated by Clare Southby-Tailyour with later additions by David Glenister.

Date	Title	Archival Reference
NK	Discussion paper on 'Nursing Staff'	C305(Box4)/44

NK	A review of some of the work reported in the field of community care (Dingleton Study)	C305/1/6/2/1
NK	Perspectives on a community psychogeriatric service	C305/1/6/1/8
NK	The effectiveness of the Community Psychiatric Services provided by Dingleton Hospital for Psychogeriatric patients in the Borders	C305/1/6/1/7
NK	Evaluation of the service for psychogeriatric patients provided by Dingleton Hospital expressed by general practitioners in the Borders.	C305/1/6/1/6
NK	Guest editorial	C305/1/3/22
NK	The effects of inter-professional relationships	C305/1/1/11
NK	Relationship of nursing theory to research	C305/1/1/12
NK	A review of some of the work reported in the field of community care	C305/1/3/44
NK	Professional nursing practice in relation to research. [International Conference: 'The Reality of the Nursing profession in a Cultural Perspective'. School of Higher Education for Health Professionals]	C305/1/5/17 and C305/1/9/1
NK	Higher education and the nursing profession in Scotland	C305/2/2/4
NK	Book Review: *Technical Skills in Registered Nursing and Related Occupations* by Analie Rademoker	C305/1/8/14
NK	Book Review: *Psychiatric Care and Conditions* by E. Longhorn (2nd ed.) . Chichester: John Wiley and Sons	C305/1/8/16
NK	Book Review: *Community Nursing in Developing Countries: A Manual for the Community Nurse* by M. Byrne and F.J. Bennett	C305/1/8/24
NK	Book Review: *Psychological Care in Nursing Practice* by M.E. Hyland and M.L. Donaldson. London: Scutari Press	C305/1/8/32
NK	Book Review: *Counterblasts No.13*	C305/1/8/43
1957	*Aids to Psychiatric Nursing*. London: Balliere, Tindall and Cox	...
4-15 Nov 1957	*The nurse in the psychiatric team* [W.H.O, Copenhagen]	C 305/1/9/2

1962	*Aids to Psychology for Nurses* (1st ed.). London: Balliere, Tindall and Cox	...
1964	Group dynamics and nursing care. *International Journal of Nursing Studies* **1**, pp. 151-158	C305/1/4/17
1964	*Aids to psychiatric nursing.* London: Balliere, Tindall and Cox	...
1967	A critique of the Salmon report. *International Journal of Nursing Studies* **4**, pp. 113-117	C305/1/3/37
1968	Measurement of patient-nurse interaction in relation to in-patient psychiatric treatment. (MSc thesis)	...
1969	'Tutors away'. *Nursing Times* **65** (6) 6 February 1969 pp. 21-24	C305/1/3/39
22-27 Apr 1969	Report on a visit to Warsaw	C305/2/7/7
1969	Reflections on nursing. *Maudsley Gazette*, Autumn pp. 85-90	...
1969	*Psychiatric Nursing* (formerly '*Aids to Psychiatric Nursing*'). London: Balliere, Tindall and Cassell	...
3 Apr 1970	Patient/nurse interaction in the psychiatric scene. *Nursing Mirror*, **130** (14) 3 April 1970	C305/1/3/8
10 Apr 1970	Go and talk to the patients. *Nursing Mirror*, **130** (15) 10 April 1970	C305/1/3/49
Apr 1970	Co-operation between disciplines in the mental hospital with special reference to the nursing staff (Dingleton Project)	C305/1/6/1/1
10-13 Nov 1970	Methods and resources available for the training of nursing personnel. World Health Organisation: working group on education and Training in Long term care, including Geriatrics	C305/1/3/32
1971	Relationships between patients and nurses in psychiatric wards. *International Journal of Nursing Studies*, **8** pp. 179-187	C305/2/7/5
1972	*Patient-nurse interaction; a study of interaction patterns in acute psychiatric wards.* Edinburgh: Churchill Livingston	...

Jul 1972	Study of the multidisciplinary approach to psychiatric treatment provided at Dingleton Hospital in the Scottish Border counties with particular emphasis on the nurse's role	C305/1/6/2/4
2 Nov 1972	Small group teaching and the joint education of architects and education. Raman P.G. and Altschul A. *Art* 2	C305/1/3/15
Feb 1973	Nursing and Social Work: A look at the Briggs Report. *Focus* Feb	C305/1/4/18
19 Apr 1973	A multidisciplinary approach to psychiatric nursing. *Nursing Times*, **69** (15) 19 Apr 1973	C305/1/4/1
5 Feb 1973	Reviews of visits to patients in September 1972 (Dingleton Project)	C305/1/6/1/2
Jul 1973	Study of the multidisciplinary approach to psychiatric treatment provided at Dingleton Hospital in the Scottish Border counties with particular emphasis on the nurse's role. Part Two	C305/1/6/2/5
9 May 1974	Beginning and end. *Nursing Times* **70** (19) 9 May pp. 718-9	C305/1/5/51
1973	*Psychiatric Nursing* (4th ed.). London: Balliere Tindall	...
13 Jan 1977	Interview: Annie Altchul. *Nursing Times*, 13 Jan pp. 50-51	...
21 May 1977	The use of nursing care plans or the implementation of the nursing process in psychiatric nursing. [Wessex Regional Conference of the Association of Nursing Education, Salisbury]	C305/1/1/14
2 Sep 1977	Education and Role of Nurses. [139th Annual Meeting of the British Association for the Advancement of Science, University of Aston.]	C305/1/1/15
8 Sep 1977	Use of the nursing process in psychiatric care. *Nursing Times* 8 Sep pp. 1412-1413	C305/1/3/7
8 and 15 Sep 1977	Professing Nursing [Inaugural Lecture. Delivered on 10 May 1977, University of Edinburgh]. *Nursing Mirror* **145** (10) pp. 7-9 (part 1) [8 Sep] *Nursing Mirror* **145** (11) pp. 27-30 (part 2) [15 Sep]	C305 (Box 4)/9
1977	*Psychiatric Nursing* (5th ed.) Altschul A.T. and Simpson R. London: Balliere Tindall	...

1977	'RCN Code of Professional Conduct: A discussion document' Dawson J.D., Altschul A. and Sampson C. *Journal of Medical Ethics* 3 pp. 115-123	C305/1/3/35
21 Feb 1978	'Twenty one years of Nursing Studies at Edinburgh', Altschul A.T. and Tierney A.J. *University of Edinburgh Bulletin* 14 (7) 21 Feb	C305 (Box4)/37
11 May 1978	Bachelors and masters of nursing. *Nursing Mirror*, 146 (19) pp. 7-8 11 May	C305 (Box 4)/42
25 May 1978	Education and the role of nurses. *Nursing Times* 74 (21) pp. 885-887 25 May	...
Jul 1978	A measure of education. *Australian Nurses Journal* 3 (4) pp. 885-887, Jul	...
Jul 1978	Scotland: University of Edinburgh Department of Nursing Studies. *Journal of Advanced Nursing* 3 (19) pp. 388-390	...
1978	A systems approach to the nursing. *Journal of Advanced Nursing* 3 pp. 333-340	C305/1/3/40
1979	Commitment to Nursing. [Battersea Memorian Lecture, 3 Nov 1978]. *Journal of Advanced nursing* 4 pp. 123-135	C305/1/1/17
26 Apr 1979	Jumping ahead with Jay. *Nursing Mirror* 148 (19) pp. 17-19, 26 Apr	...
28-29 Jun 1979	The Responsibilities of the profession in relation to change. [The Queen's Institute Scotland Conference: District Nursing and Health Visiting- Taking Stock.] *District Nursing Newsletter*, Nov 1979	C305/1/1/18
1 Nov 1979	Progress relating to the mental health nurse in his/her care for the mental health of the community. 5th Convention of the Australian Congress of Mental Health Nursing, Perth.	C305/1/1/19
1980	*Multiple choice questions: book 3: psychology for nurses: pharmacology for nurses* by R.E. Baily. London: Balliere Tindall	...
1980's	Myths, legends and fairy tale endings. *Community Care: Life begins at 40?* A review of attitudes towards community care since the post-war period. [Perth]	C305/2/2/18

13 Mar 1980	Psychiatry under review part 1. The care of the mentally disordered: three approaches. *Nursing Times* 76 (11) pp. 452-454, 13 Mar 1980	C305/1/4/2
27 Mar 1980	Psychiatry under review part 2. The Role of Professionals. *Nursing Times*, 76 (13) pp. 555-556, 27 Mar 1980	C305/1/4/4
10 Apr 1980	Psychiatry under review part 3. Hints on maintaining patient-nurse interaction. *Nursing Times*, 76 (15) pp. 40-41, 10 Apr 1980	C305/1/4/6
1 May 1980	Psychiatry under review part 8. The team approach to psychiatric care. *Nursing Times*, 76(18) pp. 797-798, 1 May 1980	C305/1/4/9
1980	*Issues in Psychiatric Nursing: Recent Advances in Nursing.* Edinburgh: Churchill Livingstone	C305/1/2/1
26 Jun 1980	Nursing: profession, semi-profession or non-profession [Association of Administrative Psychiatric Nurses, Donegal]	C/305/1/1/13
8-12 Sep 1980	Ideas for research. [International Congress: Psychiatric Nursing for the Eighties]	C305/1/1/20
22 Jan 1981	One nurse's week. Professor Annie Altschul describes a week in her working life. *Nursing Mirror*, 22 Jan 1981	C305(Box 4)16
9 May 1981	Health teaching: A nursing activity. Nursing Studies Association Study Day [Nursing Studies Association Study Day]	C305/1/1/1
27 May 1981	A conceptual framework for psychiatric nursing	...
May 1981	The problems of safeguarding the community's interest if students are doing research. *Journal of Advanced Nursing*, 6 pp. 231-241	...
Jul 1981	Collaborative mechanism on higher education in nursing [International Workshop, San Fransisco]	C305/1/1/3.
21 Oct 1981	The 0-5 year old mentally handicapped child; from the nursing viewpoint. *Nursing Mirror* 153, (17) pp. 32-33, 21 Oct	...
3 Nov 1981	Nursing in ferment	C305/1/1/4.

1982	'The development of research in nursing', in *The Research Process in Nursing* D. Cormack (Ed.). 1st ed. London: Blackwell Scientific	C305/1/2/2
21-22 Apr 1982	Issues in psychiatric nursing, [Conference: Issues in Nursing, London]	C305/1/1/5
22 Oct 1982	The consumer's voice: nursing implications [Winifred Raphael Memorial Lecture, London]. *Journal of Advanced Nursing*, **8** pp. 175-183	C305/1/1/6a-6b.
Oct 1982	Rights for mentally ill patients. *Nursing Mirror*, **6** pp. 62-3	C305/1/3/43
1982	Book Review: To enhance (promote, advance, dignify) life; from women who care to nursing care by Marie-Francoise Collier. Paris: Inter Editions. *Journal of Advanced Nursing*, **10** 3	C305/1/8/17
1982	The effectiveness of the Community Psychiatric Services provided by Dingleton Hospital for psychogeriatric patients in the Borders	C305/1/1/7
1982?	Pathways of patient's careers: a study of findings from the study of case notes. (Dec 1981- Mar 1982)	C305/1/6/1/5
22 Feb 1982	Nursing Mirror Column (reconstruction of the nursing profession)	C305/1/7/26
22 Mar 1982	Nursing Mirror Column (nursing qualifications)	C305/1/7/23
16 Apr 1982	Nursing Mirror Column : Pass the education buck. *Nursing Mirror* 12 May 1982	C305/1/7/22
12 May 1982	Nursing Mirror Column	C305/1/7/21
4 Jun 1982	Nursing Mirror Column (continuing education for nurses)	C305/1/7/20
13 Jul 1982	Nursing Mirror Column (specialist vs. generalist)	C305/1/7/19
6 Aug 1982	Nursing Mirror Column (specialisation)	C305/1/7/18
3 Sep 1982	Talking points at conference. *Nursing Mirror* 29 September p. 48	C305/1/7/17
4 Oct 1982	Nursing Mirror Column (responsibility, conscience and personal commitment)	C305/1/7/16

28 Oct 1982	Nursing Mirror Column (university cutbacks)	C305/1/7/15
24 Nov 1982	Nursing Mirror Column (on old newspapers and journals)	C305/1/7/14
21 Dec 1982	Nursing Mirror Column (industrial dispute)	C305/1/7/13
1983	Book Review: *Research into Nurse Education*, Bryan Davis (ed) Kent: Croom Helm	C305/1/8/15
31 Jan 1983	Nursing Mirror Column (committees)	C305/1/7/12
21 Mar 1983	Nursing Mirror Column (HFA2000)	C305/1/7/11
29 Mar 1983	Psychiatric Nursing in Great Britain. [National Congress of Psychiatric Nurses, Madrid]	C305/2/2/38
22 Mar 1983	Nursing Mirror Column (training and retaining nursing staff)	C305/1/7/10
28-30 Mar 1983	Psychiatric Nursing in Great Britain. [2nd National Congress of Psychiatric Nursing, Madrid]	C305/1/1/8
14 Apr 1983	Nursing Mirror Column : The alarm bells are ringing. *Nursing Mirror* **156** (20), 18 May p. 31	C305/1/7/9
20 May 1983	Nursing Mirror Column (General Election)	C305/1/7/7
20 Jun 1983	Nursing Mirror Column (relationships between doctors and nurses)	C305/1/7/6
5 Jul 1983	Nostalgia for the Good Old Days: Whose Interest is Served? [University of Edinburgh 4th Centenery Celebration. Department of Nursing]	C305/1/1/9
13 Jul 1983	With all due respect: why relations with medical and nursing staff seem to have reached such a low ebb. *Nursing Mirror* 13 Jul	C305(Box 4)/17
13 Jul 1983	Nursing Mirror Column (ritual and ceremony)	C305/1/7/5
8 Aug 1983	Nursing Mirror Column (National Boards/UKCC)	C305/1/7/4
5 Sep 1983	Nursing Mirror Column (NHS cuts)	C305/1/7/2
29 Sep 1983	Nursing Mirror Column (services for the elderly)	C305/1/7/3
1983	Book Review: *Research into Nurse Education*, Davis B.D (ed) Kent: Croom Helm. *Medical Education* **18** (5) Sep	C305/1/3/42

1983	Nursing and higher education. *International Journal of Nursing Studies* **20** (2) pp. 123-130	C305/1/3/31
1983	The thistle and the edelweiss (interview with Alison Morton). *Nursing Mirror* **157** (2) pp. 18-19	...
1983	Critique of *Psychology and Nursing: the case of an empirical approach*, L. Wattley and D. Muller. *Journal of Advanced Nursing* **8** pp. 335-342	C305/1/4/16
1983	Book Review: *Nursing 1*, D. Middleton. *British Book News*	C305/1/8/11
1983	Book Review: *Ladies without Lamps*, Eve Williams, London: Thomas Harmsworth Publishing. *Journal of Advanced Nursing*	C305/1/8/23
2 Nov 1983	Farewell Annie (interview with Jane Salvage). *Nursing Times* 79 (44) 2 Nov pp. 10-12	...
Jan 1984	Psych nursing In Great Britain. *Journal of Psychosocial Nursing* 22 1	C305/1/5/50
1984	A comparison of *Balliere's Nursing Dictionary* and Oxford Medical Publication's *Pocket Dictionary for Nurses*	C305/1/3/16
11 Jul1984	Does good practice need good principles? Part One. *Nursing Times* **80** (28) 11 Jul pp. 36-38	...
18 Jul 1984	Does good practice need good principles? Part Two. *Nursing Times* **80** (29) 18 Jul pp. 49-51	...
18 Jul 1984	A challenge to psychiatry. *Nursing Times* **80** (29) 11 Jul pp. 49-51	...
25-27 Sep 1984	The conference in perspective. [*Nursing Times* Conference-From Hospital to Home]	C305/1/5/13
10 Oct 1984	Safe journey home. *Nursing Times*, **80** (41) 10 Oct pp. 18-19	...
11-13 Nov 1984	An Overview of the British and European Approach to Theory Development in Nursing. [75th Jubilee Celebration, University of Saskatoon]	C305/1/1/10
1984	Book Review: *Depression*, D.P.B Goldberg, Edinburgh: Churchill Livingstone	C305/1/8/18

1985	*Psychiatric Nursing: a concise nursing text*, (eds.) A. T. Altschul and M. McGovern. Edinburgh: Churchill Livingstone	...
1985	Book Review: *Patient Assessment in Psychiatric Nursing*, Philip Barker. *Journal of Advanced Nursing*	C305/1/8/10
1985	Book Review: *The Nursing Process in Psychiatric Nursing*, Felicity Stockwell	C305/1/8/9
1985	Book Review: *Whose Body Is It?*, Caroline Faulder, London: Virago Press	C305/1/8/7
1985	Book Review: *Assessment and Intervention in Geropsychiatric Nursing*, Celeste Dye, Orlando: Grune and Stratton. *Journal of Advanced Nursing*	C305/1/8/12
1985	Book Review: *Ageing: recent advances and creative responses* , A. Butler (ed) British Association of Gerontology, Kent: Croom Helm	C305/1/8/40
1985	Book Review: *Psychiatric Nurse Therapists in Primary Care*, I. M. Marks, London: Royal College of Nursing. *Journal of Advanced Nursing*	C305/1/8/41
1985	Book Review: *Psychiatric Nursing Skills: A patient-centered approach*, G. Dexter and M. Walsh. London: Croom Helm. *British Book News*	C305/1/8/42
25-26 Sep 1985	Nursing research and education. [International Congress, Vienna]	C305/2/2/3
25-26 Sep 1985	Nursing research for better care. [International Congress, Vienna]	C305/2/2/2
22 Nov 1985	Nurse training. [Once an Institution, Always an Institution- residential care for Mentally Handicapped People]	C035/2/2/1
13 Feb 1986	The last decade in psychiatric nursing: what does it hold for the next? [Shropshire Psychiatric Institute]	C305/2/7/8
Mar 1986	The elderly make the world go round. *Geriatric Nursing*, 6 (2) Mar/Apr 1986 pp. 26-7	C305(Box 4)/32
30 Jul 1986	Branching out- project 2000. *Nursing Times*, **82** (31) 30 Jul, 1986 pp. 47-48	C305(Box 4)/7

24 Sep 1986	Mental health nursing: the voice of realism (interview with Martin Vousden). *Nursing Times*, **82** (39) 24 Sep pp. 26-27	...
1986	Book Review: *Florence Nightingale and the Nursing Legacy*, Monica Baly*British Book News*	C305/1/8/13
1986	Book Review (joint): *Models for Nursing*, B. Kershaw and J. Salvage, Chichester: Wiley and Sons.*Building and Using a Model for Nursing*, S. Wright, London: Edward Arnold. *Journal of Advanced Nursing*	C305/1/8/19
1986	Book Review: *Behavioural Therapy- Maudsley Book of Clinical Management*, Bristol:, Wright. *Journal of Advanced Nursing*	C305/1/8/20
1986	Book Review: *Learning to Care in Community Psychiatric Nursing*, M. Ward and R. Bishop, London: Hodder and Stoughton. *Journal of Advanced Nursing*	C305/1/8/21
1986	Book Review: *International Issues in Nursing Research*, S. M. Stinson and J.C.Kerr (Ed.) London: Croom Helm. *Journal of Advanced Nursing*	C305/1/8/28
1986	Book Review: *Psychology and Psychiatry: an integrated approach*, P. Dally and M. Watson, London: Hodder and Stoughton.	C305/1/8//22
1987	'Specialisation in nursing'. L. Hockey (1987) (ed) *Recent advances in Nursing: Current issues*, Edinburgh: Churchill Livingston. pp. 76-89	C305/1/2/3
1987	'Why higher education for nurses? Issues and developments'. *Nurse Education Today*, 7 pp. 10-16	C305/1/3/9
16 Sep 1987	'Evaluation of Scottish Examination Systems', H. C. Sinclair and A. T. Altschul. *Nursing Times*, **83**(37) 16 Sep p. 48	C305 (Box 4)/30
1987	Book Review: *People with Mental Handicap; perspectives on intellectual disability*, J. Hatterslet, G.P. Hosking, D. Morrow and M. Myers, London: Faber and Faber. *Journal of Advanced Nursing*	C305/1/8/26
1987	Book Review: *Dealing with Drugs; helping the drug taker*, Annas Dixon, London: BBC Books	C305/1/8/227
1987	Book Review: *Depression*, Robert Romanis, London: Faber and Faber	C305/1/8/28

1987	Book Review: *Psychiatric Nursing; a therapeutic approach*, P. Martin (Ed.) Basingstoke: Macmillan. *Journal of Advanced Nursing*	C305/1/8/35
1988	Book Review (joint): *Nursing elderly people: the growing base of knowledge*, S.J. Redfern, D. Cormack, J. Brooking (Eds). *Ageing and Society*, **8** pp. 85-94	C305/1/3/13
1988	Der alte verwirrte Patient und seine Pflege in der Germeinde. *Pflege*, **1** pp. 44-49	C305/1/3/14
1988	Further Care: a study of moves from sheltered housing into long-stay care. Bield Housing Association	C305/1/6/1/4
1988	Book Review: *Symptoms of the Mind; an introduction to descriptive psychopathology*, Andrew Simms, London: Balliere Tindall. *Journal of Advanced Nursing*	C305/1/8/25
1988	Book Review: *Changing Futures; housing support services for people discharged from psychiatric hospitals*, D. Braisby, R. Echlin, S. Hilland, H. Smith-King, London: King Edward's Hospital fund for London. *Journal of Advanced Nursing*	C305/1/8/29
1988	Book Review: *Psychiatric and Mental Health Nursing; a commitment to care and concern*, J. E. Perko and H.Z. Kreigh, London: Prentice Hall International (UK).	C305/1/8/31
1988	Book Review: *Human Behaviour in Illness*, (4th ed.) L. Gillis, London: Faber and Faber	C305/1/8/32
1988	Book Review: *Psychiatric and Psychosocial Perspectives*, L. Paine (Ed.) Kent: Croom Helm. *Journal of Advanced Nursing*	C305/1/8/39
1989	Book Review: *Family Therapy in the Community*, Duncan MacPhail, Oxford: Heinemann Professional Publishing.*Journal of Advanced Nursing*	C305/1/8/8
1989	Book Review: *Depression; an integrated approach*, K. Herbst and E. Paykel (Ed.) Oxford: Heinemann Medical Books.*Journal of Advanced Nursing*	C305/1/8/30
1989	Book Review: *Stress and Coping in Nursing*, R. Baily and M. Clarke, London: Chapman and Hall. *Journal of Advanced Nursing*	C305/1/8/33

1989	Book Review: *Mental health and Psychiatric Nursing*, L. Aromando, Pennsylvania: Springhouse Corporation. *Journal of Advanced Nursing*	C305/1/8/34
1989	Book Review: *Nursing Elderly People*, C. A. Dye (Ed.) Edinburgh: Churchill Livingstone. *Journal of Advanced Nursing*	C305/1/8/44
1989	*Student assessment in basic nursing education in Scotland*, A. T. Altschul, H. C. Sinclair. *Nurse Education Today*, **9** pp. 3-12	C305/1/3/11
1989	A qualitative analysis of examination questions set for students of nursing in Scotland, A. T. Altschul, H. C. Sinclair. *Nurse Education Today*, **9** pp. 161-171	C305/1/3/12
1989	One or many? *Community Psychiatric Nursing Journal*, Dec pp. 14-18	C305/1/3/41
2-3 Feb 1990	The consumer perspective. [RCN Conference, Perth]	C305/1/5/12
Oct 1990	The future in trust in trust: a response to the UKCC's discussion paper on post-registration education and practice. *Community Psychiatric Nursing Journal*, **10** (5) pp. 14-17	...
1990	Psychiatric and mental health nursing. *Journal of Advanced Nursing*	C305/1/8/6
1990	Foreword to *Fear Not to Sow: A Life of Elsie Stephenson.* Penzance: Jamieson Library	...
1990	Book Review: *The place of special villages and residential communities. Journal of Advanced Nursing*	C305/1/8/4
1990	Book Review: *An evaluation of very sheltered housing. Journal of Advanced Nursing*	C305/1/8/36
1990	Book Review: *Medical Quotations*, J. Dainith and A. Isaacs. London: Collins Reference Dictionary. *Journal of Advanced Nursing*	C305/1/8/37
1991	Book Review: *Community Psychiatric Nursing - The 1990 National Survey. Journal of Advanced Nursing*	C305/1/8/5
1991	Book Review: *Principles and Practice of Psychiatric Nursing*, S.G. Wiscarz and S.J. Sundeen, St. Louis: Mosby. *Journal of Advanced Nursing*	C30/1/8/46

1991	Book Review: *Psychiatric Nursing Audit: a study of practice*, R. Balough. Carlisle: Garlands Hospital. *Journal of Advanced Nursing*	C305/1/8/38
1991	Book Review: *We Can Speak for Ourselves*, P. Williams and B. Schoultz, London: Souvenir Press. *Journal of Advanced Nursing*	C305/1/8/45
1991	Book Review: *Under the Weather: Alcohol Abuse and Alcoholism: how to cope. Journal of Advanced Nursing*	C305/1/8/47
1991	Book Review: *Basic Behaviour Therapy. Journal of Advanced Nursing*	C305/1/8/48
1992	Book Review: *Effective Approaches to Patients' Behaviour* G.B. Lipkin and R.G. Cohen, New York: Springer Publishing. *Journal of Advanced Nursing*	C305/1/8/49
1992	Book Review: *Comforting the Confused: strategies for managing dementia*, S.B. Hoffman and C.A. Platt, New York: Springer Publishing. *Journal of Advanced Nursing*	C305/1/8/50
1992	Book Review: *Perspectives in Gerontological Nursing*, E.M.Baines, London: Sage Publications. *Journal of Advanced Nursing*	C05/1/8/53
1992	Is British nursing education jumping out of the frying pan and into the fire? *Journal of Advanced Nursing*, 17 pp. 1391-1392	C305/1/3/34
1992	Book Review: *Families of Schizophrenic Patients; cognitive behavioural intervention*, C. Borrowclough and N. Tarrier, London: Chapman Hall. *Journal of Advanced Nursing*	C305/1/8/54
1992	Book Review: *Understanding Dementia* by A. Jacques. Edinburgh, Churchill Livingstone. *Journal of Advanced Nursing*	C305/1/8/55
1992	Book Review: *Women and Mental Health- Challenging Stereotypes*, M. Barnes and N. Maple, Birmingham: Venture Press. *Journal of Advanced Nursing*	C305/1/8/56
1992	Book Review: *Normalisation in the 90's. Journal of Advanced Nursing*	C305/1/8/57
1992	Book Review: *Primary Health Care and Psychiatric Epidemiology*, B. Cooper and R. Eastwood, London: Routledge. *Journal of Advanced Nursing*	C305/1/8/58

1993	*Experiences of a hip replacement.* ? Churchill Livingstone	C305/1/3/48
1993	Book Review: *Models for Mental Disorders: Conceptual Models in Psychiatry*, 2nd (Ed.) P. Tyrer and D. Steinberg, Wiley and Sons, 1993	C305/1/3/30
1994	*Altschul's psychiatric and mental health nursing*, A.T. Altschul	...
1994	Book Review: *Reshaping Dementia Care; practice and policy in long term care*, M.K. Aronson, California: Sage Publications	C305/1/8/51
1994	Book Review: *Medical Knowledge: doubt and certainty*, C. Seale and S. Pattison (Eds.) Buckingham: Open University Press. *Journal of Advanced Nursing*	C035/1/8/52
Aug 1995	Editorial comment. A. T. Altschul and T. Butterworth. *International Journal of Nursing Studies*, **32** (4) pp.339-340.	...
1995	Book Review: *Precursors and Causes in Development and Psychopathology*, D. Hay and A. Angold (Eds.) Wiley and Sons, 1993. Blackwell	C305/1/3/29
Jan 1996	(with other contributors) Janforum: a celebration of 20 years of scholarship in nursing, midwifery and health visiting: the first 20 years of the Journal of Advanced Nursing. *Journal of Advanced Nursing*, **23** (1) pp.3-10	...
Jun 1996	Foreword to *Altschul's Psychiatric and Mental Health Nursing*. London: Balliere Tindall (1994)	C305/1/8/3
Dec 1996	Guest editorial. *Journal of Psychiatric and Mental Health Nursing*, **3** (6) Dec p.345	...
Dec 1996	Nurses who work with mentally disordered people should be appropriately qualified. *Journal of Psychiatric and Mental health Nursing*, **3** (6) p.45	...
1996	Book Reviews: *Five books concerning child psychiatry. Journal of Psychiatric and Mental Health Nursing*, **3** pp. 1-5	C305/1/3/38
1996	Book Review: *My Fifty Years in Nursing- Give us to go blithely*, D.R. Schwarz, Springer, 1995. Blackwell Science Ltd (1996)	C305/1/3/36
11 Mar 1996	A personal view of psychiatric nursing	...